AIDS & Adolescents

by Linda Thayer

Introduction by
Bernard Cardinal Law

ISBN: 0-8198-0744-3

Printed in the U.S.A. by St. Paul Books & Media
50 St. Paul's Avenue, Boston, MA 02130

Contents

Introduction

In November 1989, the Pontifical Council for Pastoral Care of Health Workers organized an international Conference on AIDS which was held in the Vatican. Participating in that meeting were many of the most important figures involved in the AIDS crisis, including those credited with isolating the virus and those who were doing the most research on it around the world. There were care providers and activists who joined political and religious leaders of every type and background to examine the issue and see what responses would best respond to this modern pandemic.

These were not men and women who shared one religious faith or one philosophy or ideology. There was no restriction on what they wished to say. In fact there was a wide variety of opinions expressed on almost every aspect of this major, modern challenge. In all the diversity of opinion and discussion, there was one conviction everyone shared: the key to reversing this tide would be found only in modification of human behavior patterns.

The material that is offered to you in this study goes far to demonstrating the truth of that conviction. Ultimately the only adequate response to the prevention of AIDS and the elimination of sexually transmitted diseases lies in the behavior of human beings, men and women like you and me, who have to reflect on how they act and take responsibility for their actions. Whatever be a person's thoughts about certain devices – and this study raises some fundamental warnings about placing trust in devices – the real problem at issue is human behavior.

This work is offered as an attempt to underscore the fact that our efforts today must focus on the centrality of human behavior. In the long history of humanity there always have been and always will be men and women who make choices that are unhealthy and even life threatening. The Church will always seek to help them in whatever ways it can. The Church has a long history of care for those in need and it certainly will respond with love and compassion to those who are stricken by the AIDS virus.

The Church also knows that mercy must be joined to truth and that true compassion must offer to everyone the best choices possible.

Because of this commitment to accompany every human being on the pilgrimage of life, the Church is especially concerned about young people in our society today. When a spokesperson from the Boston Bureau of Student Health and Development tells us "kids know a lot about AIDS and HIV prevention but it hasn't translated into behavioral changes," then we know it is time to take a second look at the proposals that are receiving the most media attention and publicity. A careful look at what is being offered and the results of those programs can lead to only one conclusion: "value free" sex education courses that teach you about "safe or safer sex" do not do the job.

By contrast, sex education courses that stress abstinence and are geared to a teenager's cognitive and emotional level can and will make the lives of young people free from the fear of unwanted pregnancy and sexually transmitted disease. They also will make for happier, more wholesome young men and women in every other way. The Archdiocese of Boston has been offering these kinds of courses on sex education in its Catholic schools for years. It has instituted a comprehensive AIDS education program that for the last two years has proven successful in its aim of educating about AIDS in a manner consistent with sound attitudes about human sexuality and human choices.

The answer lies ultimately in behavior. Can we adults encourage responsible behavior patterns and support those behavior patterns by the education and guidance that are needed to reinforce them? I think we can. I know we can. The Archdiocese of Boston is publishing the following study with that aim: to offer to our society and especially young men and women the possibilities of programs that will encourage the best in them and support them as they mature so that they will be able to make judgments about their future free of the pressures that a culture of selfish egoism tries to press upon them.

It is my hope that everyone truly interested in a better future for the young men and women of our society will read this study. It presents wholesome and positive ways to communicate those values which are basic to better personal and family lives. This study rests on a respect for and confidence in young people, and on the conviction that the young can live by moral principles when these are fairly presented.

Bernard Cardinal Law
Archbishop of Boston

Chapter One

Why Aren't Today's Programs Working?

Since AIDS was first diagnosed in 1981, nearly 200,000 Americans have developed this disease; 64% of these have died.[1] An estimated 1 to 1.5 million others carry the human immunodeficiency virus, HIV, most of them unaware yet still capable of transmitting it to others,[2] primarily through sexual intercourse or intravenous drug abuse. 4,514 cases of AIDS have been diagnosed in Massachusetts as of November, 1991, 39% of whom reside in the City of Boston;[3] 25 to 35 thousand Massachusetts residents are estimated to carry HIV, again, most of whom are unaware, yet capable of transmitting the disease.[4] AIDS has touched every segment of society, regardless of age, race or sex. HIV can be transmitted from a mother to her unborn child; at present over 3,000 children under the age of 13 have been diagnosed with AIDS, 100 of them in Massachusetts.[5] Although Blacks and Hispanics comprise less than 16% of the U.S. population,[6] 45% of AIDS patients are members of these communities, most of which have fewer resources available to cope with the costs of treatment and care.[7] And, although the highest percentages of transmission occur among homosexual and bisexual males, and intravenous drug abusers, anyone can be at risk for AIDS through the exchange of body fluids with an infected partner.[8]

Response to the AIDS epidemic has centered around three areas of concern: research to find a cure and/or treatment for those with AIDS; testing, counseling and medical care for AIDS patients; and prevention of further spread of the disease. Perhaps the only "hopeful" aspect of the AIDS epidemic is that contracting the disease is

100% preventable, with education being considered the key to prevention strategies.

Recently, much of the public's attention has been drawn to the spread of HIV among adolescents. Although a relatively small number of 13-19 year olds have been diagnosed as having AIDS (751),[9] it is important to remember that the latency period of the disease—the time from acquiring the infection to the expression of symptoms of the illness—averages from 8 to 10 years.[10]

Currently, AIDS patients between the ages of 20 and 29 comprise 20% of the total,[11] which means that most of them acquired HIV as adolescents. Other data suggests that adolescents, and particularly low income and urban adolescents, may be the next group to experience a dramatic increase of the spread of HIV. Several indicators of this concern were reported recently in the *New York State Journal of Medicine* and are summarized below.[12]

Groups Tested	**HIV +**
Military Screening	1.4/1000
College Health Services Attendees	2.0/1000
Job Corps Applicants	3.9/1000

Because the Job Corps largely serves urban youth, 16-21, who are unemployed and out of school, the data suggests that low income and urban adolescents may be at greater risk than the general adolescent population. Furthermore, statistics, particularly those from New York City, indicate an alarming pattern for a possible AIDS explosion among adolescents:

- 60% of white urban females have had intercourse by age 19; 80% of black urban females have had intercourse by age 19;[13]
- New York City accounts for 20% of all reported cases of AIDS among 13-21 year olds in the U.S;[14]
- AIDS has become the 7th leading cause of death among people aged 15-24;[15]
- the national rate of HIV infection is 1.6/1000; the rate for the Bronx and Manhattan is 16/1000;[16]

• 8% of adolescents at a center for runaway and homeless youth in New York were tested and found to be HIV positive—this included 15% of 19 and 20 year olds.[17]

Earlier this year, the New York City Board of Education voted to confront the potential expansion of the AIDS epidemic in the adolescent population by distributing condoms in high schools without the knowledge or consent of parents.

In Massachusetts, the Board of Education and many others have also called for the distribution of condoms to high school and junior high school students as the most appropriate response to the AIDS epidemic; many have called once again for the establishment of school-based clinics and/or contraceptive education and referral systems as a solution to both the spread of AIDS among adolescents and to address the issue of teenage pregnancy; many have even called for these responses without the awareness or consent of parents.

At first glance, these may seem like positive steps, a ready remedy to the spread of a deadly virus, and a means of reducing teenage pregnancy. It is tempting to focus on a seemingly easy and available prescription to the spread of AIDS; it is tempting to live with the illusion that since we have done something, we have therefore done the best that we could. However, now is the time to ask the most critical questions and shape public policy accordingly. Now is the time to ask:

1) Will condom distribution stop the spread of AIDS among adolescents?
2) What are the effects of adolescent contraceptive programs?
3) Have these programs reduced teenage pregnancy?
4) Are there other alternatives? How effective are they?

Evaluation of available data, research regarding the effectiveness of condom use, and the negative impact of contraceptive education and services for adolescents of necessity lead to opposition to these solutions for the following reasons:

1) distribution of condoms will not stop the spread of AIDS among adolescents, whether homosexual or heterosexual;
2) condom distribution will generate a false sense of security

among adolescents with respect to a fatal disease;

3) the provision of contraceptive services for adolescents has been accompanied by increased rates of adolescent sexual activity, STD's, and teenage pregnancy, rather than a reduction;
4) school-based clinics which refer for, prescribe or dispense contraceptives have failed to reduce teenage pregnancy.

By contrast:

1) abstinence programs for adolescents, including inner-city adolescents, have been demonstrated to be effective; and
2) parental involvement in issues of adolescent sexuality, values education, and school achievement have been demonstrated to be most effective in reducing early sexual activity, teenage pregnancy and potentially, the spread of AIDS.

Ineffectiveness of Condom Use

Failure rates for the use of condoms to prevent pregnancy are well known and well documented. In evaluating the effectiveness of condoms for use by adolescents to prevent the spread of AIDS, two factors must always be kept in mind. First, failure rates given for pregnancy prevention are based on two variables—the fertility of the woman and the success of the condom as a barrier to the passage of semen. In order for the AIDS virus to be transmitted, the first variable can be dismissed; it is not relevant to the transmission of the AIDS virus. Human fertility ranges from 6 to 10 days per cycle; therefore when the fertility factor is eliminated, any failure rates given may represent only 21 to 36% of actual condom failure in providing a barrier to the passage of semen; actual failures may be 3 to 5 times higher.

Secondly, adolescents have been consistently documented as poor users of contraceptives. As noted by the Allan Guttmacher Institute, "For most methods, women under 22 are about twice as likely to experience contraceptive failure as are those 30 and older....

12% of those [unmarried teenagers] who *always* use contraception do so [experience a contraceptive failure]...women with annual family incomes under $10,000 are two to four times more likely to experience a failure."[18] Some specific failure rates for condoms are given in Table A.

TABLE A

Condom Failure

Rate	Statement/Source
9.8-18.5%	Harlap, S., et. al., "Preventing Pregnancy, Protecting Health: A New Look at Birth Control Choices in the United States," the Alan Guttmacher Institute, 1991, p. 35.
14-16%	Jones, E., and Forrest, J., "Contraceptive Failure in the United States: Revised Estimates from the 1982 National Survey of Family Growth," *Family Planning Perspectives,* 1989, 21:3, p. 103, 109.
12% per yr.	U.S. Dept. HHS, "Your Contraceptive Choices For Now, For Later," *Family Life Information Exchange*, Bethesda, MD.
10.8%	Percentage of single women who have an unplanned pregnancy within first year of contraceptive use; condom.
18.4%	Percentage of single women who have an unplanned pregnancy within first year of contraceptive use, by contraceptive intention, under 18 (to prevent pregnancy). (Grady, et. al., "Contraceptive Failure in the U.S.: Estimates from the 1982 National Survey of Family Growth," *Family Planning Perspectives*, Vol. 18, No. 5, Sept.-Oct., 1986, p. 204, 207.)
10-20%	"Condom-user failure rates range from 10 to 20%. The condom can break, spilling semen into the vagina.... The condom can slip off and spill semen into the vagina...." (McCoy, K. and Wibblesman, C., *The New Teenage Body Book*, The Body Press, Los Angeles, 1987, p. 210.)

10%	"Condoms have a 10% failure rate in preventing pregnancy and the protection they provide against AIDS could be considerably lower...." (Seligman, J. and Gesnell, M., "A Warning to Women on AIDS," *Newsweek*, August 31, 1987, p. 12.)
3-15%	"The failure rate ranges from 3 to 15%. This is often due to failure to use condoms properly, but sometimes the products leak or break." (Kolata, G., "Birth Control: For Those Concerned with the Pill's Risk, A Look at the Choices," *New York Times Health*, January 12, 1989.)

Condoms will be even less effective among those who engage in anal intercourse. In a publication of the U.S. Department of Health and Human Services entitled "Condoms and Sexually Transmitted Diseases...Especially AIDS," the former U.S. Surgeon General C. Everett Koop, is quoted as follows:

> "Condoms provide some protection, but anal intercourse is simply too risky a practice." [19]

The publication then goes on to say:

> "Condoms may be more likely to break during anal intercourse than during other types of sex because of the greater amount of friction and other stresses involved. Even if the condom doesn't break, anal intercourse is very risky because it can cause tissue in the rectum to tear and bleed. These tears allow germs to pass more easily from one partner to another."[20]

In the September 18, 1987 edition of *U.S.A. Today*, the former U.S. Surgeon General emphasizes again, "You would expect a great many more failures in rectal intercourse than you would in vaginal intercourse, and it's important to know that."[21] Other researchers have expressed the same concern; as noted in the *British Medical Journal,* there is "no evidence that the standard condom membrane will stand up to anal sex."[22] Specific research has indicated that failure rates are in fact high among male homosexuals (see Table B).

TABLE B

Condom Failure Among Homosexual Men

Rate	Statement/Source
26%	11% of condoms ruptured and 15% of them slipped during 200 acts of anal intercourse between 17 homosexual couples. (Wegersna and Oud., "Safety and Acceptability of Condoms for Use by Homosexual Men as a Prophylactic Against Transmission of HIV During Anogenital Sexual Intercourse," *British Medical Journal,* July 11, 1987, p. 94.)
30%	"Dr. David Cohen, Director of Disease Control at the Denver Disease Control Service, reported a high rate of condom breakage among gay men participating in a CDC sponsored longitudinal study of risk reduction. About 30% of men reporting condom use in anal sex had experienced at least one instance of breakage in the previous six months. Most noticed breakage in the first 5 minutes, but one-third only after withdrawal." (Pollner, F., "Experts Hedge on Condom Value," *Medical World News,* August 28, 1988, p. 60.)

Other research has documented *the failure of consistent condom usage in preventing the transmission of the AIDS virus.* In one study, the seroconversion rate was 10%,[23] one in ten; later, it was revised upward to 17%,[24] one in six (see Table C).

TABLE C

Condom Failure Among Consistent Users

Rate	Statement/Source
10%	As an indication of the poor effectiveness of condoms as a barrier to infection, 1 of the 10 spouses who reported regular use of condoms became infected with the AIDS virus. (Fischl, M., M.D., "Evaluation of Heterosexual Partners, Children and Household Contacts of Adults with AIDS," *Journal of the American Medical Association,* Vol. 257, February 6, 1987, p. 640-644.)

17% The seroconversion rate was 17%, or one in six. (Goerdent, J. M.D., "What Is Safe Sex?" *New England Journal of Medicine,* Vol. 316, No. 21, p. 1339-1342, May 21, 1987.)

In the previously mentioned publication from the Department of Health and Human Services regarding condom use, a warning is given to users at least 10 times throughout the booklet that "condoms are not 100% safe."[25]

Furthermore, the following detailed guidelines and instructions for most effective use are also included:

- store properly;
- read the label to check for disease prevention claim;
- pay attention to expiration date on condoms with spermicide;
- use a water-based lubricant;
- be cautious about vending machines—are they exposed to extreme temperatures?
- do not keep in wallet or purse more than a few hours at a time;
- don't keep condoms in a glove compartment;
- don't open package with teeth, sharp nails or scissors;
- when you open the package, be sure you can see what you are doing;
- check to see if the condom is gummy or sticks to itself;
- check the tip for brittleness, tears and holes;
- don't unroll the condom to check it;
- beware of drugs and alcohol since they may cause forgetfulness or affect one's ability to use the condom properly.[26]

With as many as 83% of 14 and 15 year olds reporting that their first experience with sexual intercourse was unexpected,[27] (or even under other circumstances) how many of these directions can reasonably be expected to receive adolescent attention?

With so many difficulties with condoms—failure to prevent pregnancy, failure in actual use among homosexuals, failure to guarantee total protection against the AIDS virus both in the lab and among well-motivated users, the high number of directives for optimum protection – **aren't we encouraging adolescents to gamble with death by distributing condoms in schools?**

National Impact of Family Planning Services for Adolescents

In the past, the Allan Guttmacher Institute, research arm of Planned Parenthood, has estimated that family planning clinics would avert between 200 and 300 teenage pregnancies per 1000 clients. Millions of dollars were spent at federal, state and local levels to fund these services in the hope of achieving this stated goal. How successful has this approach been? What are the implications of this policy for stopping the spread of AIDS among adolescents?

In the fall of 1986, Joseph Olsen and Stan Weed of the Institute for Research and Evaluation in Salt Lake City published a study which statistically analyzed the data available to determine if in fact these programs had reduced the incidence of teenage pregnancy. What they found was that although expenditures climbed from $11 million dollars annually in 1971 to $442 million dollars in 1981, and although the involvement of adolescents in clinic programs rose from 300 thousand to 1.5 million teenagers, the rate of teenage pregnancy also rose from 95 per thousand in 1972 to 113 per thousand in 1981; the number of abortions rose from 190,000 in 1972 to 430,000 in 1981. The researchers drew the following conclusions:[28]

1) there was a net increase of 50 to 120 *pregnancies* per 1000 teenage clients;
2) there were 30 fewer live *births* for every 1000 teenage clinic clients; and,
3) enrollment in a family planning program appeared to *raise* a teenager's chances of becoming pregnant and having an abortion (Olsen and Weed, see Figure 1).

FIGURE 1

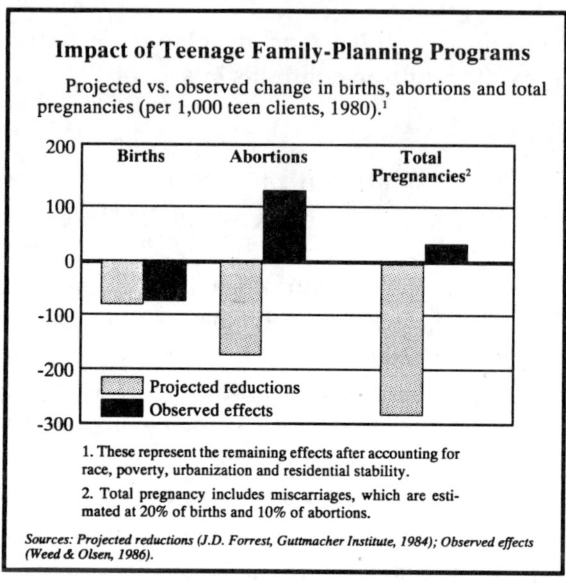

From the *Wall Street Journal,* October 14, 1986.

In fact, overall, acceptance or advocacy of contraceptive use to teenagers has been associated with a higher likelihood of adolescent intercourse in other studies as well. Also in 1986, Harris and Associates published the results of a survey conducted on behalf of Planned Parenthood. Among the questions asked of adolescents in the study were the following:

1) Have either of your parents ever talked with you about sex and how pregnancy is caused, or not?
2) Have your parents, or any other adult in your family *ever* talked with you about using birth control methods, or not?

Among those teenagers who have had intercourse, nearly half of them, 47%, were teenagers whose parents had discussed the use of birth control with them. A similar percentage, 46%, was found among those students who had "comprehensive" sex education in school.[29] Since adolescents in the study indicated that fear of disease, impact of pregnancy on one's future and parental reaction would be the most influential reasons for convincing teens to delay intercourse (65%,

62% and 50% respectively), and since the use of birth control would seemingly eliminate these reasons, it is not surprising that **parental or adult acceptance or advocacy of birth control is associated with a greater likelihood of teenage sexual activity.**[30]

Several studies have demonstrated that prior contraceptive education increases the chance of initiating intercourse among female adolescents and increases the frequency of intercourse as well.

- prior contraceptive education was shown to increase the odds of starting intercourse at age 14 by a factor of 1.5;[31]
- exposure to programs that either distributed contraceptives or told adolescents where to obtain them was "positively and significantly associated with the initiation of sexual activity at ages 15 and 16," increasing the odds by a factor of 1.2;[32]
- studies of clinics in Los Angeles and Illinois revealed that providing contraceptives to sexually active females increased their sexual activity by a factor of 1.5.[33]

Impact of Six School-Based Clinics

At the present time, there are over 178 school-based clinics, located in 32 states, serving middle junior and high school students.[34] Recently, an evaluation of six of these clinics attempted to measure the impact of such programs on sexual behavior, contraceptive use and pregnancy rates. The six clinics were located in low income areas; at five of the six clinics, the majority of the students were black; the clinics were located in Gary, San Francisco, Muskegon, Jackson, Quincy and Dallas. Some of the findings are summarized below:

Pregnancy Rates

1) **none of the clinics had a statistically significant effect on school-wide pregnancy rates; clinic presence was not associated with lower rates of pregnancy at any of the sites** (p. 6, 14).
2) overall, 1/4 of the pregnancies occurred *after* the students had obtained contraceptives from the clinic (p. 14).
3) some teenagers who conceived while in high school subse-

quently dropped out and were not present to complete a questionnaire (p. 9). (This may mean that pregnancy rates actually *increased.*)

Contraception

1) **providing contraceptives on site was not enough to significantly increase their use (p. 6).**
2) there was no indication that sexually experienced students were more knowledgeable about pregnancy prevention or more comfortable with contraceptive use than students in comparison schools (p. 14).
3) a substantial portion of female students who obtained birth control pills either did not return to the clinic for subsequent cycles of pills or did not return in time to allow continuous contraceptive coverage for six months or more (p. 11).
4) sexually experienced students were asked if they ever had intercourse without using a contraceptive method and, if so, why? The two most commonly identified reasons were "didn't expect to have sex" and "just didn't think pregnancy would occur" (p. 13).

Two additional factors were not given evaluation and are most important in assessing the impact of these programs prior to making public policy decisions regarding schools, pregnancy, contraceptives and AIDS prevention:

1) what percent of female students in these programs dropped out of school due to pregnancy; and,
2) what percent of adolescents in these programs *always* used contraceptives to protect against disease or prevent pregnancy?

First, as the authors of this clinic assessment concede, "Some teenagers who conceived in high school subsequently dropped out and were not present to complete a questionnaire."[35] The number of dropouts would be significant in assessing the impact on pregnancy. In one adolescent program in Baltimore, the loss of females was three times higher in the schools which referred for contraceptives than in the comparison schools.[36] Unfortunately, this most recent study of school-based clinics did not assess the impact of the clinic on the dropout rate among female students, nor determine how many females may have dropped out due to pregnancy. Therefore, the possibility of clinic presence increasing the pregnancy rate may still be open.

Second, in the surveys, students were asked if they had used a contraceptive method at *last* intercourse; they were not asked if they *always* used a contraceptive method during intercourse. Assuming that condoms provide 100% protection against HIV transmission, an individual adolescent's protection against AIDS depends on perfect use each and *every* time he/she has intercourse. No determination was made as to what percentage of adolescents served by the clinics were "always-users."

Another study of adolescents was conducted in San Francisco to determine if increased awareness of the AIDS epidemic impacted their use of condoms. The authors reported as follows:

> Over a year when public health information regarding AIDS intensified, changes in perceptions and use of condoms in a sample of sexually active adolescents in San Francisco were examined. Although perceptions that condoms prevent sexually transmitted diseases (STD's) and the value and importance placed on avoiding STD's remained high, these were neither reflected in increased intentions to use condoms nor in increased use. Only 2.1 percent of the females and 8.2 percent of the males reported using condoms every time they had intercourse during the study year.[37]

The Lesson of the 80's

None of the above findings regarding the overall and specific failures of contraceptive programs for adolescents are new; documentation of the ineffectiveness of these programs has been consistent in the literature throughout most of the past decade (see Table D).

TABLE D

Adolescent Use of Contraceptives

Year	Statement/Source
1983	Over a 15-month period, 6 out of 10 young adolescent patients who got a contraceptive at a family planning clinic failed to use it consistently. Since these young women, as part of a special study, received more than the usual amount of follow up, it is probable that the discontinuation rate among most clinic patients is even higher. (Furstenburg, et. al., "Contraceptive Continuation among Adolescents Attending Family Planning Clinic," *Family Planning Perspectives,* 15:211, 1983.)
1984	"Within one year after getting a prescription method from a clinic, one of eight teenage patients becomes pregnant; within two years, the fraction is nearly one out of four. Among black clinic patients, the record is even more dismal; two in ten get pregnant within a year and four in ten do so within two years. The fact remains that attending a family planning clinic and obtaining a prescription method there fails to prevent a subsequent pre-marital pregnancy among a substantial proportion of adolescent patients." (Lincoln, R., "Clinic Teenagers' High Pregnancy Rate," *Medical Tribune,* May 22, 1984.)
1985	"For most methods, women under 22 are about twice as likely to experience contraceptive failure as are those 30 and older...12% of those (unmarried teenagers) who always use contraception do so (experience a failure)... women with annual family income under $10,000 are two to four times more likely...to experience a failure." *(Issues in Brief,* Vol. 5:4, the Allan Guttmacher Institute, January 1985, p. 2, 3.)
1985	Manpower Demonstration Research Corporation concluded, after a study completed in New York, Boston, Phoenix and Riverside, California, that while increased access to contraceptives was said to have produced "promising" preliminary results in reducing teen pregnancy, later results showed that this reduction was transitory. One

year after leaving the program, teenagers had the same pregnancy rate as those who had never enrolled. *(New York Times,* May 19, 1985.)

1985 "Continued patient compliance (in contraceptive use) poses a real challenge to health clinic practitioners. Many adolescents fail to use continually and properly a method of birth control even after they have obtained that method.... frequent contact with contraceptors is important." (Kirby, D., et. al., "School-Based Clinics: An Emerging Approach to Improving Adolescent Health and Addressing Teenage Pregnancy," Center For Population Options, p. 8.)

1986 The Young Parent Program at Children's Hospital has found that "increased accessibility of birth control does not significantly alter the second pregnancy rate in adolescents. Although extended counseling on contraception is an integral part of this program, and 50% of all patients reportedly use oral contraceptives after a first pregnancy, the program showed a repeat pregnancy rate of 17.9%, compatible with the national average...." (Birth Control Access Not Factor in Teen Repeat Pregnancy Rate," *Ob-Gyn News,* January 1-14, 1986.)

1986 Researchers at the Family Planning Council of Southeastern Pennsylvania report that teenagers given "intensive follow-up" and other "special services" had the same cumulative 15-month pregnancy rate (about 13%) as the control group which had simply received contraceptives at a clinic. (Hercog-Baron, et. al., "Supporting Teenagers' Use of Contraceptives: A Comparison of Clinic Services," *Family Planning Perspectives,* Vol. 18, No. 2, March-April 1986, p. 61-66.)

1986 The percentage of single women (under 18, intending to prevent pregnancy) who have an unplanned pregnancy within the first year of contraceptive use, by method: Pill, 11.0%, IUD 10.5%, Condom 18.4%, Diaphragm 31.6%, Spermicides 34.0%. (Wm. Grady, et. al., "Contraceptive Failure in the U.S.," *Family Planning Perspectives,* Vol. 18, No. 5, Sept.-Oct. 1986, p. 207.)

1988 In San Francisco, "over a year when public health information regarding AIDS intensified...perceptions that condoms prevent sexually transmitted disease and the value and importance placed on avoiding STD's remained high, [but] these were neither reflected in increased intentions to use condoms nor in increased use" by adolescents. (Kegeles, S., et. al., "Sexually Active Adolescents and Condoms: Changes Over One Year in Knowledge, Attitudes and Use," AJPH 78:4, 1988, p. 460.)

1991 "Providing contraceptives on site was not enough to significantly increase their use...none of the clinics had a statistically significant effect on schoolwide pregnancy rates...a substantial proportion of young women did not obtain cycles of pills from the clinics often enough to allow continuous coverage...." (Kirby, D., et. al., "Six School-Based Clinics: Their Reproductive Health Services and Impact on Sexual Behavior," *Family Planning Perspectives,* Vol. 23, No. 1, Jan.-Feb. 1991, p. 6-16.)

The reasons for failure in use of contraceptives are many, varied and complex; most, if not all, simply cannot be resolved by merely counseling, referring for or distributing contraceptive devices. Serious study of underlying adolescent issues must be undertaken and more appropriate and successful programs be established accordingly.

Underlying Issues

Advocates of contraceptive services for adolescents frequently attribute the high rate of teenage pregnancy to lack of access to contraceptives for adolescents; they cite cost, availability and confidentiality as major obstacles. In this view, reducing cost, increasing availability and providing confidentiality would be sufficient to increase contraceptive use among adolescents and thereby reduce unintended pregnancy (and prevent the spread of AIDS). However, among sexually active teens who do not always use contraceptives themselves, these factors have been shown to be of minor concern; they are more of a reflection of adult concerns, rather than those of adolescents. According to the Harris Survey conducted for Planned Parenthood and published in 1986, access, cost and parental reaction were not cited as major prohibiting factors by inconsistent or non-contracepting sexually active adolescents.[38] In percentages, only

1% cited cost
3% cited embarrassment or fear
2% didn't know where to get them
4% were afraid of parental reaction
5% didn't know enough about them and
6% couldn't get them

The single greatest individual reason given was unexpected sex, 21%. For a variety of reasons 39% did not want to take time or preferred not to use them.[39] These findings were further reinforced in the recent analysis of the impact of six school-based clinics serving low income and predominantly black teenagers. Sexually experienced students who did not consistently contracept were asked why. The two most commonly identified reasons were "didn't expect to have sex" and "just didn't think pregnancy would occur." *Most of the reasons were not related to access to contraceptives, but to the fact that sex was not anticipated, to perceptions of low risk of pregnancy or to questions of motivation,*" and most importantly, as the authors report, *"clinic presence did not appear to reduce any of these reasons."*[40]

Many girls, 69% in the Harris Survey, pointed to fear of a pelvic exam as a barrier to pill use; agreement was given by 70% of those girls who have actually used the pill themselves, and presumably had undergone a pelvic exam. Fear of the exam was not removed by having a prior exam itself.[41]

It is clear that merely addressing factors of cost, access and confidentiality of services will be insufficient to either decrease the incidence of adolescent pregnancy or stop the spread of AIDS. Rather than concentrating on adult perceptions and concerns with respect to contraceptives, it would be more beneficial to examine three areas of adolescent sexual activity and pregnancy which still remain largely unregarded and unaddressed:

1) the psychological development of adolescents;
2) adolescent valuation of pregnancy;
3) underlying factors associated with adolescent sexual activity and pregnancy.

These factors must be acknowledged before shaping a public policy with respect to adolescents, contraceptives and AIDS.

Psychological Development of Adolescents

Psychological development during adolescence includes establishing an adult identity and sense of individuality, separating psychologically from the family, developing operational thinking, and planning for the future.[42] Classic understanding of adolescent development makes a clear distinction between modes of thought in adolescence and those of mature adulthood. Adolescents function at a developmental level of *concrete operational thought,* characterized by a failure to anticipate future outcomes and the haphazard processing of information; mature adults function at the level of *formal operational thought,* characterized by anticipating and weighing future outcomes, and associating behavior accordingly.[43] The two factors most essential to mature sexual decision-making and consistent use of contraceptives – anticipating and evaluating future outcomes, and associating behavior accordingly – are not fully developed during adolescence. Lack of recognition of the intrinsic nature of adolescents' cognitive skills – concrete operational thought – is one main reason why so many contraceptive programs for adolescents have failed to achieve their goal. Many researchers have begun to acknowledge the importance of this aspect of adolescent development and its relationship to teenage sexual activity, pregnancy, and potentially to the spread of AIDS:

> "There is no correlation between advanced biological maturation and cognitive development...the cognitive development of

adolescents may not permit them to comprehend fully the consequences of their behavior. To understand that sexual behavior may lead to pregnancy requires anticipation of consequences of behavior...the infrequency and spontaneous nature of early sexual activity make effective contraception problematic and increase the risk of adolescent pregnancy." (Elizabeth R. McAnarney, M.D., and William R. Hendee, Ph.d.)[44]

"Study of adolescent development shows that cognitive growth lags behind physical maturation. Until about the age of 16, adolescents are still using concrete thinking skills. As a result, young teenagers have limited ability to recognize the potential impact of their choices; they are less likely than older teenagers to think about the future and to consider the consequences of their actions." (Marion Howard, clinical director of the Teen Services Program at Grady Memorial Hospital)[45]

"Young teens are simply not capable of internalizing contraceptive information; young people just don't have the psychological strength to recognize the consequences of their actions. They tend to be impulsive, have trouble deferring gratification and making long-range plans." (Irma Hilton, psychologist at the Ferkauf Graduate School of Psychology)[46]

The reasons for contraceptive failure among adolescents include "ignorance or lack of cognitive maturity to understand physiological processes, contraceptive techniques and probability of pregnancy." (The Task Force on Pregnant and Parenting Teens in Massachusetts)[47]

"It may be that developmentally, younger teens are not able to effectively apply the knowledge that they have." A knowledgeable 13 year old is no more likely to use contraceptives than is an uninformed 13 year old. (Michael Young, in "The Planned Parenthood Poll: A Secondary Analysis of National Data")[48]

"In one study of high school students, students who were more knowledgeable about the probability of becoming pregnant did not report unprotected intercourse less frequently than those who were less knowledgeable." (U. S. Office of Technology Assessment)[49]

The implications for AIDS prevention strategies and pregnancy reduction among adolescents is clear and begins with acknowledging realities of adolescent development. Programs must be developmentally appropriate in recognition of the fact that adolescent cognitive skills differ significantly from those of mature adults. **Therefore, contraceptive education and distribution, including condoms, will be ineffective in stopping the spread of AIDS among adolescents or in reducing teen pregnancy.**

Adolescent Valuation of Pregnancy

One vital element of the teenage pregnancy problem is frequently overlooked by those who advocate contraceptive services for adolescents; a significant proportion of teenage pregnancies are on some level, deliberate and positively valued. The reasons for positive valuation of early pregnancy are varied and complex and simply cannot be resolved by providing contraceptives.

The Adolescent Resources Corporation runs three school-based clinics in Kansas City, MO. According to the director, they have teenagers who come in for a pregnancy test who are disappointed when the tests are negative.[50] According to one psychologist, pregnancy may bring attention to a girl who may be feeling neglected. For a girl who feels isolated, a baby offers the possibility of someone to love. Other girls see pregnancy as a way to assert independence from their parents or to become their mother's equal. Still other girls may see pregnancy as a way of "entrapping a reluctant suitor" or of keeping up with their pregnant girlfriends. It might also be noted that single parenthood is now more socially acceptable. Positive valuation of a pregnancy is not confined to adolescent girls; in one study, teenage fathers were generally happy about their girlfriend's pregnancy, whether or not they had any intention of caring for the child, feeling that the pregnancy had affirmed their manhood.[51]

According to the profile of these adolescents given in the report of the Task Force on Pregnant and Parenting Teenagers in Massachusetts, many adolescents saw having a baby as:[52]

- something which would "give them a sense of being needed and loved";
- a way "to get their own security and nurturing needs met";
- something which would "give them a sense of fulfillment";
- "a viable option to what their lives are" or "the only option left open to them"; or
- "a validation of an adult role" and "a way to gain some independence from their families."

In the view of many adolescents, having a baby fulfills a need for attachment or a need to be needed. Having a baby is seen as giving purpose to life or alleviating loneliness.[53] Clearly, these misperceptions and *needs of adolescents* must be recognized and addressed. Earlier identification of at-risk youth must take place and appropriate intervention strategies be developed in order to reduce these types of adolescent pregnancies. Contraceptive services are simply irrelevant to these perceptions of adolescents.

Underlying Factors Associated with Adolescent Sexual Activity and Pregnancy

Frequently, those who advocate contraception as the solution to adolescent sexual activity, pregnancy and AIDS overlook the significant numbers of teenagers for whom sexual activity and pregnancy are symptomatic of, or are associated with deep-seated psychological problems—part of a pattern of personal or socioeconomic stresses. As reported by the Massachusetts Task Force in 1986, pregnant and parenting teens included adolescents who[54]

- may have been abused as children;
- may have multiple problems themselves (drug and alcohol abuse, depression);
- exhibited low self-esteem;

- had a history of being deprived and neglected;
- had family problems.

For these teenagers, sexual activity and pregnancy were part of a much larger problem rather than a single issue requiring contraceptive services. An early assessment of school-based clinics in New York City reported a similar finding. According to the evaluation conducted by Welfare Research, Inc., and released in 1987, "Psychological problems were reported for a larger proportion of students who had used the clinic for reproductive health services than of students who had received general health care."[55] Their findings are summarized below:

	General Health Care	**Reproductive Health Care**
Family Problems	17%	35%
Depression	15%	27%
Attempted Suicide	6%	17%

Sexual activity for these students is associated with and is indicative of deep personal and emotional stresses, stresses that cannot be adequately addressed by the provision of contraceptives. A more recent study of young adolescents revealed that early sexual activity was associated with other psychosocial risks—alcohol and drug abuse, school suspension, trouble with police, etc. Sexually active girls were six times more likely to have attempted suicide than those who were inexperienced.[56] Provision of birth control devices may only serve to confirm, complicate and further accelerate an adolescent's involvement in unhealthy behaviors or destructive relationships.

Finally, as many others have noted, many of the motivations for a teenage pregnancy are born of hopelessness, the feelings that opportunities in life are few and limited; feelings that are most common among lower income teenagers who see success in school or work as impossibilities for themselves.[57] The Massachusetts Task Force has also associated teenage pregnancy with low school achievement, low aspirations and the perception of high school as pointless, removed from reality and not a step towards self-sufficiency.[58]

Teenagers who are academically behind are three times more likely to become unwed parents than those who are achieving well in school.[59] Clearly, the school's role in reducing sexual activity, pregnancy and stopping the spread of AIDS involves a much more concerted effort to diagnose underachievement at earlier ages and provide appropriate academic and remediation strategies; closer ties between academic success and a fulfilling future must be given greater clarity and attention for these students. **Any approach to reducing adolescent sexual activity, pregnancy and AIDS must be multi-faceted and simply cannot be based on contraceptive education and the distribution of condoms.**

Chapter Two

A Model That Works! The Atlanta/Emory Story

Shaping Public Policy for Adolescents

If comprehensive sex education, linked with contraceptive referrals and services, is not the solution to reducing teenage pregnancy, what is? If condom distribution and promotion will not stop the spread of HIV among adolescents, what will? What alternative strategies have demonstrated success in changing adolescent attitudes and sexual behaviors?

A Prototype of Successful Change

In the mid-70's, Emory University School of Medicine and Grady Memorial Hospital's Teen Services Program developed and implemented a comprehensive sex education program for adolescents aged 16 and under. Information covering basic human sexuality, contraceptive methods and decision-making were presented during five classroom periods; students were encouraged to seek contraceptive counseling and services. Assessment of the program by the staff revealed the following:[60]

- providing information to young teens was not effective in changing the sexual behavior of young adolescents;

- young adolescents who received the instruction were not more likely to refrain from sexual intercourse than those who had not;
- those young adolescents who had participated in the program and engaged in sexual intercourse were not more likely to use birth control than those who had not.

Research by the staff to determine why this pattern emerged indicated that **knowledge-based programs, including those with decision-making components, did not impact the health *behaviors of young adolescents.*** The educational model utilized in the program—information on human sexuality, information on contraception, and decision-making—was ineffective because it was inconsistent with the psychological development of young adolescents. Cognitive growth in adolescence lags behind physical maturation until the age of about 16. Young adolescents utilize concrete thinking skills (dealing with immediate experiences, difficulty in thinking about the future consequences of actions) as opposed to adult formal operational thought (weighing future outcomes and associating behavior accordingly). *Young adolescents were not able to effectively apply to their sexual behavior the things that they knew*—about sexuality, pregnancy and contraception. Additionally, *the role of social influences, the media and peer pressure were acknowledged as propelling young adolescents into sexual activity.* Finally, and most significantly, survey data collected by the Emory/Grady Teen Services Clinic indicated that *many young people were looking for ways to say "no!"* "Of nearly two dozen items thought to be of interest, teenage girls surveyed were most likely to indicate that they wanted more information on how to say "no" without hurting the other person's feelings (84%)."[61]

A new program was designed around strategies which:

- were appropriate to the psychological development of young adolescents;
- were designed to help students identify the origin and motivations of peer and social pressure; and

- would help students develop the skills to respond to pressure by saying "no."

Since young teens frequently want to be and act older, and since they look up to slightly older adolescents as role models, older teens would be used to present the information, role play responses to pressure, and teach assertiveness skills. This would also serve to provide evidence for young teens that those who say "no" could be admired and liked, that sexual activity is not the only way to obtain status. The program would not be lecture oriented in nature, but experiential: students would think about and discuss pressure to become sexually active and they would practice skills helpful to them in resisting peer pressure. Thus, the program was designed to meet the expressed and behavioral needs of adolescents.[62]

Implementation of a controlled study to determine the effectiveness of the program, Postponing Sexual Involvement, was undertaken during the 84-85 school year among 536 eighth graders in Atlanta. Students involved were black (99%), low-income teenagers (53%) determined to be at high risk for early sexual activity and pregnancy. The results of the comparison between program and non-program students included the following:[63]

- students who had *not* had the program were as much as *5 times* more likely to have begun having sex than those who had had the program (p. 23);
- by the end of the 8th grade, girls who had *not* had the program were as much as *15 times more likely* to have begun having sex as were girls who had had the program (p. 24);
- there were fewer pregnancies among the program group because there were fewer girls who were sexually involved; *the program appears to have reduced pregnancies by one-third* (p. 25);
- although the program was not reinforced in grade 9, by the end of the ninth grade, 39% of those who had not had the program had begun having sex compared with 24% of the program group (p. 24, Table 2);
- of all students who acknowledged having sex after the pro-

gram was offered...the program group appeared more likely only to have experimented with sex: They described themselves much more often than the no-program group as having tried sex just once or twice (43 vs. 28%)...this makes the point that just because a person has had sex, it does not mean that he or she has to continue to be sexually active (p. 24);

- to assess whether or not the students perceived Postponing Sexual Involvement as enabling them to have more control over their sexual behavior, they were asked: "With respect to the information the teen leaders or person from Grady Hospital taught, how helpful will that information be to you personally in saying no to sex?" Of the young people who had not had sex before the program, 95% said that program would be helpful to them personally in saying no to sex and more than 80% thought the program would be extremely helpful or very helpful (p. 24);
- the majority of young people in both the program and non-program groups who did have sex did not use contraceptives (p. 25);
- girls who had become sexually involved had similar pregnancy rates...corroborating previous data suggesting that the provision of human sexuality and family planning information...is not sufficient to help many sexually involved young people to avoid pregnancies (p. 25).

In light of these results, Emory/Grady Teen Services Program is currently developing a program for fifth and sixth graders aimed at helping them handle their curiosity about sexual involvement and develop attitudes and skills to manage sexual behaviors as they become young teenagers; a follow-through program aimed at reinforcing for ninth and tenth graders the information and skills they have learned in eighth grade is also being developed so that a "continuum of consistent educational messages combined with repetitive skill-building will increase the effectiveness" of the program.[64]

Despite the despair of many adults that "the kids are going to do it anyway," Postponing Sexual Involvement (and other

programs of a similar nature such as Sexuality Commitment and Family and Sex Respect) have amply demonstrated that, given proper understanding, motivation and skills, young people can be taught to resist pressure; they can be taught to abstain. The reduction in sexual activity, pregnancy and contingently STD's (including AIDS) was accomplished by:

- a critical assessment of current strategies;
- acknowledging limits and failures;
- determining need by hearing adolescents; and
- developing and implementing appropriate new strategies.

All of which culminated in a basic but profoundly far reaching reversal in strategy:

> "Although one of the major *implicit* goals of the earlier program was to assist young people in postponing sexual involvement, that goal is made *explicit* in the revised outreach approach."[65]

It perhaps bears repeating that part of the success of the Postponing Sexual Involvement Program lies with the fact that the reduction of sexual activity and pregnancy occurred among a minority, low-income, high-risk teenage population – high-risk in terms of both pregnancy and AIDS; these were the young people who resisted pressure and abstained. 61% of American teenagers say that social pressure is the chief reason why so many of their peers do not wait to have sexual intercourse until they are older; 72% of those who have had sexual intercourse agree.[66] If pressure is the major problem, what would be the impact of mass distribution of condoms to adolescents? More pressure? More sexual activity? More condom failures? More pregnancies? More STD's? And more adolescents infected with HIV? **If pressure is the main problem, then reducing pressures on young people and equipping them with tools to resist and say "no" effectively become the answers** – enabling them to take greater control of their lives, reducing sexual activity, teen pregnancy, and the transmission of AIDS.

A public policy for the 90's to reduce adolescent pregnancy and AIDS should begin with an application of the same success-producing process outlined above – assessing current strategies, acknowledging failures and limits, determining need and developing/implementing appropriate new strategies – as carefully, but as quickly, as possible. Since the preparation of this document began, an additional 27,915 Americans have been diagnosed with AIDS.[67]

Chapter Three

Condom Promotion vs. Abstinence Education

Despite claims to the contrary by those who advocate contraceptive-oriented sex education, adolescents' perceptions that adults are advocating the use of contraceptives, or that adults accept or approve of sexual activity that is "protected" are associated with higher rates of sexual involvement. This was strikingly evident in the Harris Survey conducted for Planned Parenthood in 1986. Consider the following:

A. *With respect to topics covered by parents with adolescents:*

TABLE E

Parental Conversations

Topic	**% of Adolescents Who Have Had Intercourse**
Sex, pregnancy, using contraceptives (339)	49% (165)
Neither subject (284)	35% (98)
Sex, pregnancy only (312)	27% (84)

** Calculations based on data, page 45, "American Teens Speak: Sex, Myths, TV and Birth Control."

B. *With respect to adolescent perception of parents' wishes regarding use of contraceptives:*

TABLE F

Parent's Wishes Regarding Contraception

Parents Wishes Regarding Birth Control	% of Adolescents Who Have Had Intercourse
Would want them to use (631)	44% (277)
Would not want them to use (85)	29% (25)
Would not want them to use/not sure (179)	20% (35)

** Calculations based on data, p. 46, "American Teens Speak: Sex, Myths, TV and Birth Control."

C. *With respect to content of sex education in school:*

TABLE G

Content of Sex Education

Content	% of Adolescents Who Have Had Intercourse
Comprehensive sex education (347)	46% (161)
No sex education (371)	32% (119)
Sex education (223)	30% (67)

** Calculations based on data, p. 53, "American Teens Speak: Sex, Myths, TV and Birth Control."

(Comprehensive sex education was defined as containing four of the six following sex education topics:

- biological facts about reproduction;

- talk about coping with sexual development;
- information about different kinds of birth control;
- information about preventing sexual abuse;
- facts about abortion;
- facts about where to get contraceptives.

In this study, 2/3 of comprehensive programs cover information about birth control; 1/2 included facts about where to get them.)

Additionally, as shown in a previous section, **adolescents have been acknowledged as being consistently poor users of contraceptives (see Table D); but when they perceive, or are led to believe, that various methods are effective or will be effective for them in preventing pregnancy, levels of sexual activity are in fact higher, regardless of method.**

TABLE H

Adolescent Perceptions of Birth Control Effectiveness & Rates of Having Had Intercourse

Method/Perceived Effectiveness	**% of Adolescents Who Have Had Intercourse**
Pill	
Works well (672)	40% (270)
Not well, not sure, not familiar with (275)	28% (77)
Condom	
Works well (543)	43% (231)
Not well, not sure, not familiar with (401)	30% (119)
Diaphragm	
Works well (315)	47% (147)
Not well, not sure, not familiar with (633)	33% (207)

IUD	
Works well (202)	44% (88)
Not well, not sure, not familiar with (746)	36% (266)
Foams, Creams, Etc.	
Work well (184)	48% (88)
Not well, not sure, not familiar with (770)	35% (266)
Withdrawal	
Works well (160)	44% (70)
Not well, not sure, not familiar with (784)	36% (280)
"Safe Time"	
Works well (157)	43% (67)
Not well, not sure, not familiar with (794)	36% (284)

** Calculations based on data, p. 34-35, "American Teens Speak: Sex, Myths, TV and Birth Control."

Clearly, impressing upon adolescents a perception of optimum clinical effectiveness of any method will only contribute to increased rates of sexual activity.

AIDS Knowledge – Does It Impact Behavior?

With regard to AIDS education and adolescent awareness, a similar pattern is beginning to emerge. Education which presents knowledge regarding HIV/AIDS and condom use alone fails to impact behavior at best and accelerates rates of sexual activity at worst. Research conducted at the University of Maryland revealed the following: [68]

- 95% of students knew about AIDS prevention; yet a majority of students continued to practice high-risk behaviors;

- 68% of those who had engaged in anal intercourse continued to do so; 27% continued the practice, but less frequently;
- 56% of students who had intercourse with prostitutes continued to do so; 37% continued to do so, but less frequently.

The researchers concluded, "We found knowledge is reasonably high, yet there is little personalization of risk or behavior change due to AIDS."[69] A similar pattern was recently presented with respect to adolescents in Massachusetts; according to Kevin Cranston, from the Bureau of Student Health and Development, "Our research has shown that 90 to 95 percent of students have information on how AIDS is transmitted and how to avoid it, but many of them aren't taking proper precautions in their personal lives." Recent surveys indicated that 51% of adolescents have engaged in sexual intercourse; 60% had not taken "precautions" to protect themselves from AIDS.[70] The pattern holds true nationally as well; knowledge about AIDS and how to avoid it is high among adolescents, but behavioral changes are few, despite the fact that:[71]

- 98% of students surveyed knew that a person can infect another person with HIV during sex; and
- 93% of students surveyed knew that a person can reduce the chance of infection by using condoms; and
- 91% of students surveyed knew that there is no cure for AIDS.

Researchers have found that "having been taught about HIV and AIDS does not have a significant and direct association with any of three behavior items (having ever had 2 or more sexual partners; having had two or more sexual partners during the last year; and always using condoms)...once knowledge and background factors are controlled for, HIV/AIDS instruction is not associated with less risky sexual behavior."[72]

Students who had been taught about HIV/AIDS were no more likely to report the "always use" of condoms than those who had not had such instruction.

TABLE I

AIDS Education/Condom Use[73]

Instruction	"Always Use"	Non/Inconsistent Use
Taught about AIDS	34.4%	65.6%
Not Taught	33.4%	66.6%

Even more frightening are indications that increasing condom promotion and advocacy to prevent AIDS is related to higher rates of adolescent sexual activity. The following points were noted in a recent study of sexual activity, condom use and AIDS awareness among adolescent males. During the period between 1979 and 1988 (the same interval which witnessed the identification of AIDS, increases in contraceptive oriented sex education and promotion of condom use) *sexual activity among metropolitan adolescent males also increased substantially:*

- the number of 17-19 year old metropolitan males who had intercourse was 15% higher in 1988 than it was in 1979;[74]
- the increase among metropolitan black males aged 17-19 who had intercourse was 23%;[75]
- condom sales increased between 1986 and 1987;[76]
- media attention to condoms went from infrequent to frequent after the Surgeon General's Report was released in 1986;[77]
- rates of sexual activity for Massachusetts' teenagers were higher in 1988 than in 1986;[78]
- the adolescents in the sample were very knowledgeable about how AIDS was transmitted;[79] but
- certain high risk sub-groups had significantly lower condom use rates than average for all teens (adolescent males who were, or whose partners were IV drug users; those who had sex with a prostitute, stranger, or someone who had had many sexual partners; or those who had multiple partners themselves).[80]

What is evident is that a decade which witnessed increases in contraceptive-oriented sex education, school-based clinics, AIDS awareness and condom promotion also witnessed increased rates of sexual involvement among adolescents as well. Although the authors point out that more than half of the sexually active males surveyed had used a condom at last intercourse, they candidly admit that "this is not necessarily a measure of consistent use, and *the question remains whether consistent condom use among sexually active teenagers can become the norm*";[81] in addition, significantly lower rates were reported among those teens behaviorally at higher risk for exposure to AIDS.

The implications of aggressive condom promotion as a public policy or educational strategy to stop the spread of AIDS among adolescents are ominous. If one accepts the conservative figure of a 10% failure rate in the use of condoms in preventing HIV transmission, and assumes that 100,000 adolescents are sexually active and use condoms, and further assumes that each is exposed to an HIV carrier, then the number of adolescents at risk would be 10,000.

100,000 x 10% = 10,000

If, however, aggressive condom promotion increases the rate of sexual activity among adolescents by 15%, increasing the number of sexually active teens to 115,000, and we still accept the conservative condom failure rate of 10%, the number of adolescents at risk for exposure to HIV would be 11,500, a net gain of 1,500 adolescents.

100,000 x 15% = 15,000 additional sexually active teens
115,000 x 10% = 11,500 teens at risk due to condom failure
11,500 - 10,000 = 1,500 additional teens at risk for AIDS

Instead of decreasing the number of teens faced with the potential for developing AIDS, a public policy of condom promotion may well result in the opposite effect – an increase. This pattern has a precedent well documented through the 70's and early 80's with regard to the impact of increased provision of contraceptives for adolescents and the subsequent increase in the number of teenage pregnancies. Between 1971 and 1981, the number of adolescents who received contraceptive services increased from 300,000 to 1,500,000.[82] During that time period the percentage of *sexually active* girls who experienced a premarital pregnancy remained relatively constant (see Figure 2). However, simply by virtue of the fact that more adolescent women were sexually active, the number of *all* adolescent women, 15-19 years old who reported a premarital pregnancy dramatically increased (see Figures 3 and 4).

FIGURE 2

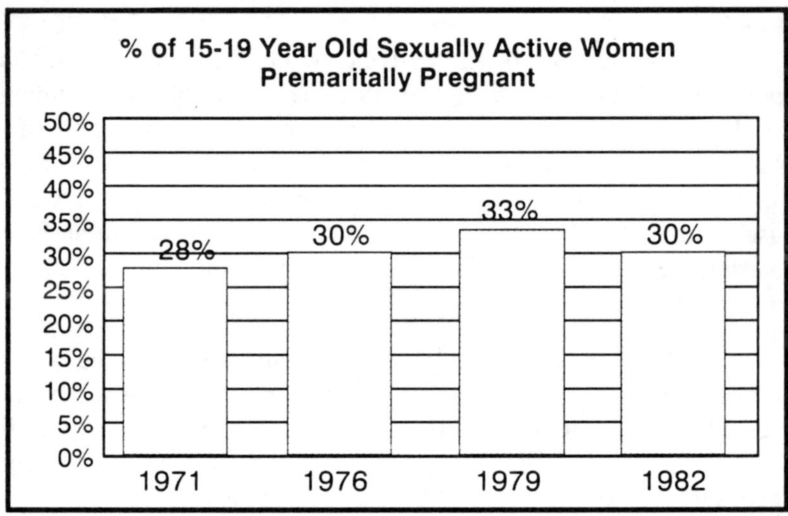

Source: Unpublished tabulations from the NSFL III; Zelnick and Kantner, 1980, Table 3 (HSC).

FIGURE 3

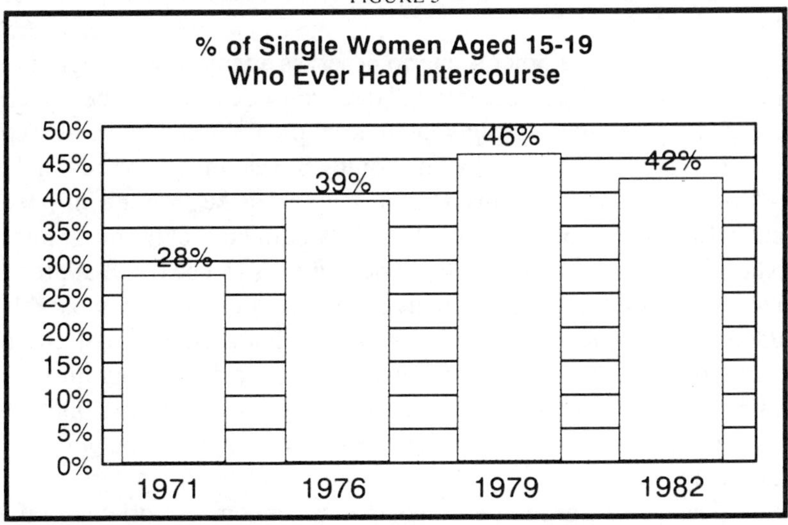

Source: Unpublished tabulations from the NSFL, Cycle III, 1982; unpublished tabulations from the National Longitudinal Survey of Youth, 1983 Zelnick'& Kantner, 1980, Table 3, (HSC).

FIGURE 4

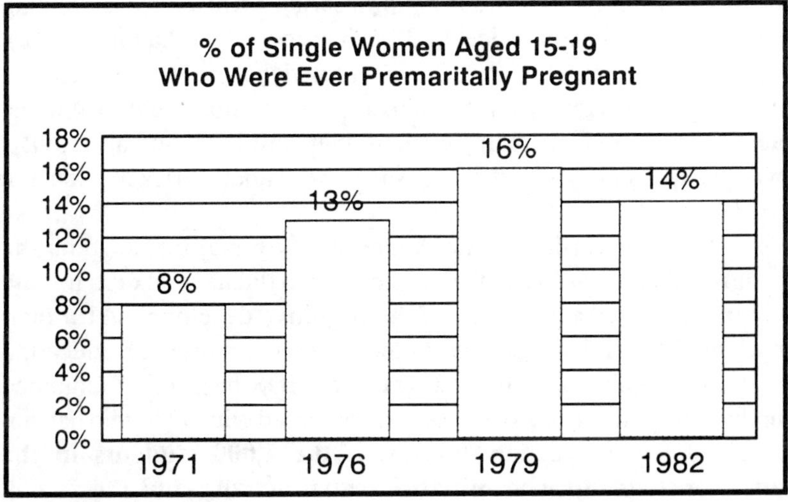

Source: Unpublished tabulations from NSFL III; Zelnick and Kantner, 1980, Table 3, (HSC).

Unfortunately, a similar pattern with respect to AIDS is just as likely.

However, one other scenario deserves attention with regard to messages given to adolescents and their consequent sexual behavior. According to percentages given in the study of the abstinence-based program piloted in Atlanta – Postponing Sexual Involvement – only 4% of the 8th grade students who participated in the program initiated sexual activity, compared with 20% of those outside of the program.[83] The positive implications of these percentages can be better appreciated by considering the two hypothetical groups of comparable adolescents – each containing 100,000 individuals. The first group participates in an abstinence-based sex education program; 4% (4000) of the adolescents initiate sexual activity, 96% (96,000) do not. A population of 96,000 adolescents remains free from potential exposure to HIV.

The second group participates in a condom-use oriented program; 20% (20,000) initiate sexual activity; 80% (80,000) do not. This time only 80,000 remain free from potential exposure to HIV. An additional 16,000 adolescents would be placed at greater risk. It may be recalled that students who participated in the abstinence program were also more likely to describe themselves as "having tried sex just once or twice" (43%) than those who had not (28%). They were also more likely to have reported that they had not had sex within the previous month;[84] meaning that adolescents from the abstinence-based program, even if they initiated sexual activity, would experience a significantly smaller cumulative risk of exposure to HIV.

As noted earlier, in the Atlanta study a majority of both the program and non-program adolescents who did have sex did not use contraceptives,[85] a reflection of the cognitive development for their particular age. It has also been noted with respect to AIDS education that 66% of students who had received AIDS instruction remained inconsistent/non-users of condoms, compared with 67% who had not received any instruction.[86] **Thus, if the 4,000 students in the abstinence group who initiated sexual activity and the 20,000 students of the condom-use group who initiated sexual activity**

used condoms in similar proportions and experienced similar failure rates, the effects of abstinence-based education would still be far-reaching, simply by virtue of the fact that substantially fewer adolescents were sexually active.

Our goal, our every effort should be aimed at guaranteeing the safety and health of *every* adolescent, protecting them from a devastating and fatal disease. The abstinence-based program conducted in Atlanta was presented at one grade level only—the 8th. Plans are currently under way to extend the program to both lower (5th & 6th) and higher grades (9th & 10th) in order to build a "continuum of consistent educational messages combined with repetitive skill-building" to increase the effectiveness of the program for adolescents.[87] Strategies for public policy should begin to do the same—employ abstinence-based strategies, as consistently and as effectively as possible in order to maximize protection for adolescents against early sexual activity, pregnancy, STD's and AIDS.

Chapter Four

Hearing What Adolescents Say

Pressure

As previously mentioned, 61% of teenagers say that social pressure is the chief reason why so many of their peers do not wait until they are older to have intercourse; among teenagers who have had intercourse, the figure is even higher — 72%.[88] Despite some of the demeaning characterizations of teenagers as "hormones with feet,"[89] only 13% of teenagers mention sexual gratification or enjoyment as a reason for having intercourse; only 8% cite being "in love" with a partner.[90]

- How pervasive is social pressure to have sex?
- How intense?
- What steps can be taken to minimize pressures and teach adolescents how to deal with it?
- What would be the impact of condom distribution on social pressure?

Nationally, 1 out of 4 high school teenagers say they personally have been pressured to "go further with sex" than they wanted to. Among those teenagers who have had intercourse, the figure is higher, 30%, nearly 1 in 3. Among black teenagers, the proportions are similar, 30%, 1 in 3. Girls are three times more likely to indicate pressure at the time of first intercourse than boys; younger teens, 12-15 years old, are more likely to cite pressure at the time of first intercourse than those who are older.[91] However, the pressures faced by young urban teenagers deemed to be at-risk — and most frequently the target of school-based clinics, or contraceptive-oriented sex education programs—may be even more intense. Based on the responses of the 536 eighth grade students involved in the analysis of the effectiveness of *Postponing Sexual Involvement* in Atlanta:[92]

- 43% of the 8th graders surveyed said they "had been alone with someone who wanted sex last month";
- 47% said they "would find it hard to say no to sex with someone they care about";
- 12% said they "never say no when asked to do something [they] don't want to do."

In addition to being in pressure situations and finding it difficult to say no, the perception of these young people as to the proportion of their peers who have had sex was substantially higher than the number who actually indicated that they had had intercourse—thus intensifying the pressure already placed on these adolescents:[93]

- 45% of the 8th grade students surveyed thought that "most (or) several of their friends have had sex";
- 41% thought that "almost everybody (or) lots of 8th graders have sex;"
- 40% thought that "their best friend has sex."

In actuality, however,

- 24% of the 8th grade students surveyed said that they had sex.

Student perceptions of the proportions of their peers who have had intercourse were nearly double the actual figure. Clearly the pressures on these adolescents were high. Promoting or distributing condoms to this population would only encourage them to accommodate the pressure to have sex, increasing their risk of pregnancy, STD's and AIDS. As previously noted, adolescents who perceive that contraceptives are effective or that "protected sex" is acceptable to adults are more likely to have had sex than those who have not (see Table H). Adolescents are also more likely to be poor or inconsistent users of contraceptives, more likely to experience a failure (see Table D). However, giving adolescents reasons for and strategies which enable them to resist pressure and say "no" have dramatically reduced the initiation of sexual activity in this population—thereby also reducing the risks of pregnancy, STD's and AIDS. Moreover, the vast majority of sexually active adolescent girls surveyed prior to the program's implementation, 84%, had indicated that *"how to say no to sexual pressure" was precisely what they most wanted to know* about sex; 95% of the students, both boys and girls, who had taken the course and had not had sex prior to it, stated that the program would be helpful to them personally in saying "no" to sex.[94]

88% of teenagers surveyed in 1986 did not think that clinics where contraceptives could be obtained should be located inside their school; 78% of black teenagers surveyed agreed.[95] Perhaps included in their reasons for this response is an unspoken acknowledgement that this would only increase the intense pressures already placed upon them.

Unexpected Sex

Nationally, 65% of teens who have had intercourse say their first experience was unexpected; 83% of 14-15 year olds say this, as well as 73% of the black adolescents in this survey.[96] Among the urban, high-risk youth surveyed in Atlanta, 43% said they "had been alone with someone who wanted sex last month."[97]

Several factors need to be considered here. First, failure to anticipate outcomes and associate behavior accordingly is an acknowledged characteristic of adolescent cognitive development. "Unexpected sex" is most likely the result of having been in a pressure situation, alone, at risk for an outcome which was unanticipated, and for which the adolescent was unprepared. "Unexpected sex" is also the reason given most frequently by teens for poor use of contraceptives.[98] Making condoms available to adolescents in this context will not resolve the problem of "unexpected sex." Of greater benefit to adolescents would be adult efforts to:

- minimize the amount of time teenagers find themselves alone and at risk;

- provide "low pressure" settings where teenagers can socialize without risk; and
- enable adolescents to effectively say "no" to early sexual activity and other high-risk behaviors.

Second, the role of drug and alcohol abuse has not received adequate attention in connection with "unexpected sex." In one recent study,[99]

- sexually experienced girls were 10 times more likely to have used marijuana and 6 times more likely to have used alcohol than those who were not;
- boys who were sexually experienced were 6 times more likely to have used alcohol and 5 times more likely to have used marijuana than those who were not.

Sexually active young teens are far more likely to have engaged in other unhealthy behaviors than those who have not. Provision of contraceptives at school is once again unlikely to impact the outcome of a high risk situation for which the adolescent was unprepared and/or is compounded by the influence of drugs or alcohol; condom distribution may serve to validate unhealthy or destructive behaviors. However, a program which enables adolescents to say "no" effectively to one high risk behavior may just as likely enable them to say "no" to other high risk behaviors as well.

Third, while some have pointed out that poor teenage utilization of contraceptives "suggests a repeated and continuing lack of anticipation on the part of many teenagers," they have failed to correlate this pattern as being characteristic of adolescents at a particular stage of cognitive development; instead, blame is placed on the adolescent for using "unexpected sex" as an "excuse or cover-up for...failure to prepare for something that should and could have been anticipated" and "a cultural tradition that discourages any combination of 'planning' with 'romance.'"[100] The latter assertion is *inaccurate;* 68% of teens in the same survey disagreed with the idea that "using birth control is unromantic because it means a person has planned to have sex in advance."[101] The former assertion is *unfair,* blaming adolescents for behavior patterns consistent with their level of maturity.

Rather than "blaming" them, **the greatest service provided to adolescents would consist in minimizing the risk situations in their lives and enabling them to take greater control of their lives by resisting social pressure placed upon them.**

Effective Arguments for Waiting

In the Harris Survey, teens were asked which arguments might be most likely to influence other teenagers to wait to have intercourse until they are older. The three top responses were,[102]

- concern about diseases, such as herpes and AIDS, 65%;
- impact of a pregnancy on one's life, 62%; and
- concern over parental reaction, 50%.

What these adolescents were saying is that three powerful, natural incentives in their lives exist which will help them postpone sexual activity. What would be the impact of condom distribution on these natural understandings of teenagers? Condom distribution would effectively cancel these incentives for postponing sexual activity by promising "freedom" from disease, "freedom" from an untimely pregnancy, and "freedom" from parental awareness of sexual activity; condom distribution would only serve to increase pressures on many adolescent lives. As noted before, adolescents who perceive the effectiveness of condoms to be high are more likely to have had intercourse (43%) than those who do not (30%) (see Table H); adolescents who have had "comprehensive sex education" (contraceptive-oriented) are more likely to have had intercourse (46%) than those who have not (30%) (see Table G). This strategy can only increase pressures on teens by destroying their natural arguments for postponing sexual intercourse thereby increasing the number of adolescents who initiate sexual activity.

What Adolescents Tell Us Behaviorally

As examined in another section of this report, the factors which underlie early adolescent sexual activity, pregnancy (and risk of AIDS) can be complex and are frequently associated with emotional, psychological and family problems experienced by the adolescent. A striking example of this was recorded in the assessment of the early school-based clinic experience in New York City. Students who visited the clinic for "reproductive health care services" were twice as likely to indicate that they were experiencing family problems, twice as likely to indicate feeling depressed and three times as likely to have attempted suicide than those who had visited the clinics for general health care.[103] Additionally, the average age of first intercourse for young adolescent women in detention centers in New York City was 12 years of age, compared with a national average age of 16 years at first intercourse.[104] Sexually active young teens are far more likely than those who have never had sex to practice an array of other unhealthy or destructive behaviors.[105] In one study, it was found that:

- sexually experienced girls were 5 times more likely to have been suspended from school and 10 times more likely to have used marijuana;
- girls who have had sex were 6 times more likely to have tried suicide;
- boys who were sexually experienced were 6 times more likely to have used alcohol and 5 times more likely to have used marijuana;
- boys who were sexually experienced were 10 times more likely to have been in a car with a drug-using driver.

Clearly, early sexual activity can be an indication of other deeply rooted problems or self-destructive behaviors.

On the other hand, an examination of the lives of adolescents who have been able to postpone sexual activity reveals another consistent pattern at work – a pattern which keeps adolescents protected against the dangers of early sexual activity, pregnancy, STD's and AIDS. This pattern involves three consistent factors: values, goals and achievement, and family environment. As Asta Kenney of the Allan Guttmacher Institute has pointed out, "the likelihood of a teenager's becoming sexually active or becoming pregnant prematurely has less to do with socioeconomic status than with the individual teen's values, goals and aspirations in life and with the kind of family environment in which he/she is raised...teenagers...who see a future for themselves are less likely to become sexually involved at an early age."[106] What is the impact of these 3 factors? Do values, goals and achievement, and family environment significantly impact adolescent sexual activity? Are they effective tools in reducing early pregnancy and the potential spread of AIDS?

Family Environment

"In shaping the values of young people, parents are more powerful than any clinic, any teacher, any peer," according to Michael Carrera, past president of the American Association of Sex Educators, Counselors and Therapists.[107] Sexuality education is a developmental process which not only involves specific discussions, factual information and values actively imparted by parents, but also the day to day experiences, relationships and observations that take place in the home. Lack of family stability has been noted by many as contributing to the problem of teenage pregnancy; the Massachusetts Task Force which studied adolescent pregnancy cited family problems, a history of feeling deprived and neglected, having been abused as a child and the perception of having a child as a way of getting their own needs met, as characteristics of many pregnant and parenting teens.[108] Adolescents who live with both parents are less likely to be sexually active than those who live with a single parent, according to Joanne Gasper, former deputy assistant secretary for Population Affairs. In the Harris Survey, 69% of high school teens living with 2 parents have not had sexual intercourse;[109] still another study has found that the presence of both parents in the home at age 14 reduced the odds of first intercourse of adolescent girls aged 14-16.[110]

Teenagers rank parents first in importance out of 11 possible sources of information about sex and birth control. Significantly, a majority of adolescents, 68%, report having had a conversation about sex and the cause of pregnancy with their parents; this includes 70% of white adolescents as well as 82% of black adolescents. 69% of teens nationally indicated that their parents were the greatest source of information about sex and pregnancy; 53% said the same was true of birth control.[111] As documented earlier, parents should be aware that the content of parental conversations with adolescents and adolescent perceptions of parental values and expectations do impact their behavior. Perceptions of the acceptability of "protected sex" and the effectiveness of contraceptives are associated with a greater likelihood of adolescent intercourse (see Tables E, F, and H).

According to adolescents themselves, three natural arguments would be compelling in helping themselves and their peers to postpone sexual intercourse — fear of disease, impact of an untimely pregnancy and concern over parental reaction. Of those who indicated concerns over parental reaction, 71% had not yet had intercourse.[112]

Values

Perhaps most striking is the impact on adolescent behavior of an active religious values system provided by parents. Several recent studies have consistently documented religious values as being a significant factor in helping adolescents abstain — thereby reducing all risks — pregnancy, STD's and AIDS:

- 79% of teenagers who attended religious services frequently have not had intercourse, compared to 56% of those who attended services seldom or never;[114]
- church attendance one or more times a week reduces the odds of first coitus for adolescent girls at all ages;[113]
- among the strongest determinants of first coitus for adolescent girls at these ages (15-16) is infrequent church attendance.[115]

Adolescents who say religion is important to them are less likely to be sexually active than those who say it is not, according to

Joanne Gasper, formerly with the Office of Population Affairs. In light of these findings, it should be the responsibility of both public policy-makers in general and school officials in particular, to acknowledge the positive role religious values play in impacting adolescent sexual activity, reducing pregnancies, STD's and AIDS. It should further be their responsibility to respect the religious freedom of parents in guiding their children in accordance with their chosen religious values. Distribution of condoms, or other school policies which contradict or subvert the religious values of parents, are a violation of the trust placed in schools by parents.

Furthermore, at least one student survey has indicated the failure of "values free" strategies to achieve the stated goal of improving adolescent decision-making. Three hundred and forty Boston Public School students in the 11th grade were surveyed in 1987; these were most likely better motivated students who survived the high dropout rates which occurs after the 9th and 10th grades. Yet, nearly half of them, 46%, indicated that their sex education courses did not help them make better decisions about their sexuality.[116] As one proponent of school-based clinics has conceded, the attempt in the past to teach sex education free of values may have been a mistake; that "all people should be treated with dignity and respect" and that "no one should use subtle pressure or physical force" in order to engage in sexual activity are basic values which should be discussed in the classroom, according to Douglas Kirby, formerly with the Center for Population Options.[117]

Although with respect to public schools the question is frequently asked, "Whose values?" the answer is perhaps not as complex as some would have us believe. While it would not be appropriate for public schools to promote the exclusive tenets or dogmas of a specific religious denomination, *it would be both appropriate, and essential* to promote those behaviors which will most effectively safeguard adolescents against early pregnancy and AIDS—abstinence and mutually faithful monogamy; it *would* be appropriate for public schools to promote those values which are common to the human experience and are regarded universally as enriching human life, despite the fact that these values may happen to coincide or overlap with religious teachings. These values might include:

- self control and restraint;
- respect for others;
- adhering to principles under pressures;
- faithfulness;
- delaying personal gratification for the sake of a greater good.

Goals and Achievements

The impact of academic achievement or failure on adolescent behavior has also received extensive documentation; adolescents who perform well in school and who have associated educational achievement with a future goal such as college are less likely to become sexually active or pregnant at an early age than those who have not.

- among those adolescents who averaged A-B+ in school, 74% have not had sexual intercourse; among those who average C-F, 57% have not had intercourse.[118]
- educational attainment at or above the expected level reduces the odds of first coitus for adolescent girls between the ages of 14 and 17.[119]
- among high school teenagers who plan to go to college, 70% have not had intercourse, compared to 56% who do not have such plans.[120]

"Older teenage females with poor basic skills are two and a half times as likely to be mothers as those with average basic skills; older teenage males with poor basic skills are three times as likely to be fathers. Among younger teens — those under 16 — females with poor basic skills are five times as likely to become mothers as those with average skills," according to Asta Kenney of the Allan Guttmacher Institute.[121]

Low aspiration, low school achievement, a belief that life offers few options and opportunities and that high school is pointless are among the characteristics of pregnant and parenting teens according to the Massachusetts Task Force study published in 1986.[122] For schools, the greatest step that can be taken to reduce the incidence of adolescent pregnancies, STD's and AIDS, is not the simplistic distribution of condoms, but increasing in each student a sense of self-esteem generated by authentic educational achievement, high expectations and the identification of goals for the future that are worth waiting for. Identification of students at risk and educational adjustments to maximize academic success and internalize a strong sense of self-worth should take place as early as possible—especially at elementary and middle school levels.

Chapter Five
Conclusions and Recommendations

An effective public education policy with respect to reducing adolescent sexual activity, pregnancy, STD's and AIDS of necessity involves a discontinuation of current ineffective sex education strategies and replacing them with those which are most medically effective, age appropriate and geared to the expressed needs of adolescents. With respect to AIDS prevention, policy makers need to begin to take seriously the failure rates in the use of condoms in preventing pregnancy (10% on average, 18% or more for adolescents) and realize the potentially higher rates of failure for preventing the spread of AIDS. The false sense of security generated by slogans of "safer sex" and "lowered risk" are potentially *life-threatening* to adolescents. Policy-makers need to begin to take seriously the assertion of the former U.S. Surgeon General that abstinence and faithful monogamy should be the *primary* recommendations to prevent the spread of AIDS.[123]

Educators need to create meaningful categories of risk among youth and adolescents and shape AIDS prevention education accordingly. According to Karen Hein, M.D., director of an adolescent AIDS program in New York City, one such group includes adolescents who are at low risk because they are "very young, are virginal, have not received blood transfusions and are not intravenous substance abusers."[124] Nationally, with respect to having had intercourse, this includes the vast majority of young adolescents. Over 90% of 7th and 8th graders, aged 12-13, have not had intercourse; 2/3 of all teenagers, aged 12-17 have not had intercourse.[125] 3/4 of the inner city

8th graders in Atlanta surveyed as part of an abstinence program had not yet had intercourse.[126] Abstinence education means promoting and maintaining the lifestyle which most teenagers already practice, and extending this message in age appropriate ways to both younger and older students.

It is also important for those who shape educational policy to distinguish in surveys between those teenagers "who have had intercourse" and those teenagers who are "sexually active." In one study, 20% of teenagers who indicated that they had had intercourse had done so only once; 42% of sexually active teenagers in a second study indicated that they had not had intercourse in the previous month.[127] 43% of the at-risk population in Atlanta who participated in the abstinence program and became sexually active had only done so once or twice; 28% of those outside the program indicated the same. Having had intercourse and being sexually active are not necessarily the same.[128] The vast majority of adolescents are already practicing a lifestyle which reduces the risk of early pregnancy, STD's and AIDS. Resisting pressures to change this lifestyle should be the key factor of educational strategies.

Based on the findings of this report and the considerations above, the following recommendations are proposed:

1) Discontinue knowledge-based sex education programs which rely on adult decision-making capabilities.
2) Discontinue "implied decision-making," with "mixed messages" that treat "abstinence as an option."
3) Promote concrete behavioral expectations which will guarantee freedom from early pregnancy, STD's and AIDS: abstinence and faithful monogamy.
4) Discontinue plans to distribute condoms and other policies inconsistent with behavioral expectations and developmental capabilities of adolescents (promoting or referring for contraceptives).
5) Present realistic information about the inadequacies of condom use as a protection against pregnancy and AIDS at appropriate age levels.

6) Equip adolescents with effective tools to resist the pressures to engage in sexual activity.

7) Present behavioral expectations consistently at all grade levels; enlist the support of parents, peers, schools, churches and media in delivering a consistent message to adolescents.

8) Provide settings in which adolescents can socialize with a reduced risk of social and peer pressure.

9) Recognize early sexual activity as a strong potential indicator of other personal, emotional or family problems and provide appropriate support services.

10) Promote values consistent with behavioral expectations; maximize student achievement; assist teenagers in identifying future goals.

For too long our adolescents have borne the consequences of an educational philosophy which sees contraceptives as the solution to teenage pregnancy, rather than enabling adolescents to tap the strength within themselves and take personal control of their lives. Sexuality education which reflects traditional values has been criticized by some who view it as nothing more than placing restrictions on the young; they have failed to see that abstinence and self control, though not without difficulties, are in fact a source of great freedom for adolescents:

- freedom from early pregnancy;
- freedom from STD's and AIDS;
- freedom from contraceptive failures and side effects;
- freedom from the trauma of an abortion decision;
- freedom from being used;
- freedom from anxiety over disappointing parents or having to "cover up";
- freedom from regret, guilt or loss of self-esteem;
- freedom to develop greater control in making life decisions;
- freedom to develop friendships rather than purely sexual relationships;
- freedom to select a life partner on the basis of love, knowledge; friendship and communication.

The time has come to acknowledge the failure of teaching adolescents to rely on contraceptive technology rather than the values and strengths within themselves; they have paid a high price in terms of abortion, disease, loss of self-worth and early pregnancy. The time has come for the adults in their lives to offer them the best alternatives and highest expectations, which will enable them to lead a more fulfilling life. Their health, their future, their very lives depend on it.

"...the threat of AIDS now confronts our generations with the end of earthly life in a way that is all the more striking because it is directly or indirectly related to love and the transmission of life...the life-giving powers of our being are in danger of becoming fatal powers" ("The Ethics of the AIDS Crisis," Pope John Paul II, September 5, 1990).

Appendix

Assessing Current Strategies

Most American teenagers have, at some point, had a sex education class at school. However, percentages receiving these courses vary. A survey of large city school districts in 1984 indicated that 80% of those districts provided some form of sex education, with 85% of the 9.3 million students receiving instruction.[129] The Harris Survey conducted for Planned Parenthood in 1986 found that 59% of American teenagers had a formal course or class in sex education at school; this included 54% of the boys and 64% of the girls.[130] However, a more recent survey of sex education teachers in 5 subject areas indicated that 93% of their schools offered sex/AIDS education.[131]

What strategies for teaching human sexuality are in place in these programs? Are they knowledge based? Do they rely on adult decision-making skills? Are they age appropriate? What messages do they promote about abstinence? ...about contraception? ...about social pressure? Some of the answers to these questions – for programs in place both nationally, at the state level, and for the Boston Public Schools – are given below.

Nationally

A. ***Knowledge-Based/Decision-Making Programs***

"Young people who had the five classes of factual and decision-making education were not more likely to refrain from sexual intercourse...nor were they more likely to use contraceptives."

Helping Teenagers Postpone Sexual Involvement

- 82-84% of sex education teachers are in schools that cover *sexual decision-making,* abstinence and birth control methods.[132]
- 90% of sex education teachers covered the topic of *sexual decision-making.*[133]
- 94% of large city school districts that provide sex education said that one of their major goals was to promote rational and informed *decision-making about sexuality.*[134]
- 77% of the districts said that their goal was to increase a student's *knowledge* of reproduction.[135]

B. "*Mixed Messages"; Implied Decision-Making; Abstinence as an Option:*

"Although one of the major *implicit* goals of the earlier program was to assist young people in postponing sexual involvement, that goal is made *explicit* in the revised outreach program."

Helping Teenagers Postpone Sexual Involvement

- 89% of teachers of sex education cover the topic of abstinence from sexual intercourse; 88% cover birth control methods.[136]
- 86% teach that abstinence is the best *alternative* for preventing pregnancy and STD's.[137]
- 92% of teachers cover abstinence as a prevention against AIDS; 91% cover condoms as prevention; 85% cover sexual monogamy as prevention.[138]

C. *Age Appropriateness*

"Study of adolescent development shows that cognitive growth lags behind physical maturation.... Young teenagers have limited ability to recognize the potential impact of their choices.... A knowledgeable 13 year old is no more likely to use contraceptives than is an uninformed 13 year old."

Helping Teenagers Postpone Sexual Involvement

- 88% of sex education teachers cover sexual decision-making in grade 7; 90% in grade 8; 92% in grade 9.[139]
- 83% of sex education teachers covered birth control methods in grades 7 and 8; 92% in grade 9.[140]
- 63% of teachers covered "safer sex" practices in grade 7 and 8; 69% in grade 9.[141]
- 87% of teachers talk to their students about negative consequences of sex for teenagers.[142]
- 66% of sex education teachers think that students should be taught about sources of birth control by the end of the 8th grade; 65% think students should be taught about "safer sex" practices; 56% think students should be taught factual information about abortion.[143]

D. *Abstinence and Faithful Monogamy*

"Abstinence and faithful monogamy with uninfected partners should be the *primary* recommendations to prevent the spread of the disease."

C. Everett Koop, U.S. Surgeon General,
International Medical News

- 75% of teachers did *not* name abstinence as their most important message.[144]
- 75% of large city districts did *not* indicate reduction of teenage sexual activity as a major goal; 60% did not indicate reduction of unwanted teenage pregnancy as a major goal.[145]
- 1% of sex education teachers say that abstinence is the only alternative for preventing pregnancy and STD's.[146]
- 9% of districts cover abstinence as the only alternative for preventing pregnancy and STD's.[147]

E. *Condom Use*

"Condoms are a *last* resort"

C. Everett Koop, U.S. Surgeon General
(U.S.A. Today, September 18, 1987)

- 77% of sex education teachers talk about how to use a condom.[148]
- 64% of teachers teach "safer sex" practices; 63% in the 7th and 8th grade; 69% in the 9th grade.[149]
- 68% of teachers encourage condom use to prevent pregnancy, AIDS, and other STD's.[150]
- 86% of districts with sex/AIDS education curricula cover using condoms as a way of preventing AIDS; 62% in the 7th grade; 63% in the 8th grade; and 64% in the 9th grade.[151]

F. *Birth Control Advocacy; Referrals; Identifying Sources For Birth Control*

"Enrollment in a family planning program appeared to raise a teenagers chances of becoming pregnant and having an abortion.... There was a net increase of 50 to 120 pregnancies per 1000 teenage clients."

Olsen & Weed; "Curbing Births, Not Pregnancies," Wall Street Journal, October 14, 1986

- 97% of sex education teachers say that sex education classes should address where students can go to obtain a birth control method.[152]
- 82% of sex education teachers will refer students seeking birth control to a family doctor; 80% will refer students to a family planning clinic.[153]
- 66% of sex education teachers believe that sources of birth control methods should be taught by the end of the 8th grade.[154]
- 52% of sex education teachers provide information about sources of birth control.[155]
- 74% of sex education teachers discuss how each contraceptive method works; 67% cover how each method is used.[156]

G. *School-Based Clinics Which Counsel For, Refer For, or Distribute Contraceptives*

"Providing contraceptives on site was not enough to significantly increase their use...none of the clinics had a statistically significant effect on school-wide pregnancy rates."

Douglas Kirby, "Six School-Based Clinics"

- currently, there are more than 178 school-based clinics operating in middle, junior and senior high schools in the U.S.[157]
- clinic services include gynecological examinations, birth control information and referral, pregnancy testing and counseling, and some dispense contraceptives.[158]
- New York City has adopted a plan to distribute condoms to senior high school students; recent editorials have advocated the distribution of condoms in the Boston Public Schools; the Massachusetts Board of Education has proposed the distribution of condoms in public schools.[159]
- a proposal for establishing school-based clinics in the Boston Public Schools was narrowly defeated in 1986; some have recently called again for establishing such clinics in Boston.

However, according to the Harris Survey conducted for Planned Parenthood in 1986:

- 88% of American teenagers do not think that clinics which provide contraceptives should be located in their schools.[160]
- 78% of black teenagers did not think such clinics should be located in their schools.[161]
- 86% of sexually experienced teenagers did not think such a clinic should be located in their school.[162]

H. *Social Pressure; Peer Pressure*

"61% of teenagers say that social pressure is the chief reason why so many of their peers do not wait to have sexual intercourse until they are older; 72% of teenagers who have had intercourse agree, as do 73% of teenage girls and 50% of teenage boys."

"American Teens Speak: Sex, Myths, TV and Birth Control"

- resistance to peer pressure for sex ranked 17th out of 24 as a topic included by large city districts.[163]

- 81% of large city districts did *not* discuss resistance to peer pressure for sex before the 9th grade.[164]
- 76% of large city districts did *not* discuss resistance to peer pressure for sex in depth (1 or more class periods).[165]
- resistance to peer pressure for sex ranked 11th out of 24 among those topics receiving one or more hours of discussion (personal values ranked first, contraceptives ranked fifth, sexual decision-making ranked seventh).[166]

AIDS Education in Massachusetts

In April of 1990, the State Board of Education approved an AIDS/HIV Prevention Education Policy for Massachusetts Schools, which urges school districts to include an AIDS/HIV prevention education program as part of a comprehensive health education and human services curriculum. At the close of the school year 1990-1991,

- 90 to 95% of students in Massachusetts had received information on how AIDS is transmitted and how to avoid it.[167]
- 87% of secondary schools across the state are providing AIDS related information to students.[168]
- 95% of school districts have designated a contact person to work with the State Department of Education to coordinate and disseminate information about AIDS.[169]
- pressure is being brought to bear on the Governor to follow through on his campaign promise regarding condom distribution in the schools.[170]

The curriculum for AIDS education in Massachusetts covers the topics of pregnancy prevention and the use of condoms to prevent AIDS; *abstinence is not specifically covered as a topic.*[171] More specifically, of 29 objectives presented in eight lessons,

- 22 objectives are concerned with HIV/AIDS information
- 6 objectives are concerned with attitudes, feelings, fears, etc.

• 1 objective is concerned with explicit decision-making.

Abstinence is merely mentioned as an option; mutually faithful monogamy between uninfected partners does not receive attention as a preventive lifestyle; "safer sex" practices and condom use receive consistent emphasis and focus as a means of prevention.[172]

According to the coordinator of the state's AIDS/HIV Education Unit, 51% of high school students have engaged in sexual intercourse; 60% have not taken precautions to protect themselves from infection with HIV. As noted by a second spokesperson, from the Bureau of Student Health & Development, "Kids know a lot about AIDS and HIV prevention, but it hasn't translated into behavioral changes."[173] – another indication that merely providing information to adolescents and assuming they have adult decision-making skills is insufficient to impact adolescent behaviors.

Sex Education and AIDS Education in the Boston Public Schools

In November of 1983, the Boston School Committee adopted the following policy with regard to sex education:

"The Boston School Committee supports the development of sex education programs in all Boston Public Schools and believes that such programs are essential to increasing students' knowledge about their growth and development and to improving their *knowledge for decision-making* in their present and future lives."[174]

This policy statement follows a philosophy in keeping with national trends in assuming that information on human sexuality and contraception, linked with a decision-making model (and local service providers) will favorably impact sexual activity, pregnancy and STD's among adolescents. This philosophy is reflected in the proposed curriculum objectives at both the middle and high school grades, ages 11-13 and 14-17 respectively. The number of objectives for each topic is given in the table below:

TABLE J

Middle School Objectives (Age 11-13)[175]		High School Objectives (Age 14-17)[176]	
4	Birth Control	6	Reproductive Anatomy and Physiology
4	Pregnancy & Birth	5	Birth Control & Abortion
3	Growth & Development	4	Sex Roles
3	Self Esteem	3	Pregnancy & Birth
3	Decision-Making	3	Relationships
2	Pregnancy Alternatives (Including Abortion)	2	STD's
		2	Homosexuality
2	Sex Roles	2	Decision-Making
1	STD's		

Careful examination of the Sex Education curriculum reveals that, in addition to explicit decision-making components, the objectives constitute an implicit but innate decision-making model which condones/promotes adolescent sexual activity and the options of birth control and abortion:

- abstinence is presented merely as a birth control option in both middle and senior high school objectives.
- local availability of birth control is explored in both the middle and senior high school objectives.
- a suggested high school activity, mentioned twice, is to invite a guest speaker from a (birth control) clinic to class.
- reading the laws regarding parental consent for abortion is a suggested activity at the high school level.
- at the middle school level, with respect to abortion, performance criteria include listing local agencies that provide counseling for pregnant minors and listing laws relating to pregnant minors.

Social pressure – the single greatest factor propelling teenagers into sexual activity – is not given status as an independent objective. Peer pressure is only mentioned within the broader context of all pressures (parents, church, TV, etc.) that "influence decision-making." At the high school level, students are asked to identify ways of counteracting "lines" used to persuade people to engage in sexual activity; but, after brainstorming all pressures, again they are asked to "apply a decision-making model," rather than practice assertive techniques in saying "no." Emphasis is not placed on abstinence, self-control and saying "no," but on "decision-making." None of the methodologies suggested with respect to peer pressure are experiential in nature; of three suggested role-playing activities in the curriculum at the high school level, and four at the middle school level, none include the experience of saying an assertive "no" to pressure. No suggestions are given as to avoiding or finding alternatives to pressure people, pressure places, or pressure activities.

With respect to the proposed AIDS curriculum, the pattern is similar; the objectives are primarily information-based, with both explicit and implicit decision-making components. Despite the assertion of the former U.S. Surgeon General that abstinence and faithful monogamy be the primary recommendations to halt the spread of AIDS, abstinence is presented as merely an option; explicit instruction in condom use is provided at all levels; mutually faithful monogamy is presented once as a topic "if there is time" at the grade 7 and 8 level. (Curriculum objectives are given in Table K.[177])

TABLE K

AIDS Curriculum Objectives

Grades 7 and 8 (12 & 13 year olds)

1. Define AIDS.
2. Explain that the cause of AIDS is a virus called HIV.
3. Identify four steps in the progression of Human Immunodeficiency Virus (HIV).
4. List the four ways through which the virus can be transmitted.
5. Name the three known body fluids through which the virus can be passed.

6. Explain how to prevent the disease and how to lessen the risk of transmission.
7. Identify hotline numbers which students can call for additional information on AIDS.

Grades 9 and 10 (14 & 15 year olds)

1. Describe the theoretical origins of AIDS.
2. Describe the history and present status of AIDS in the U.S.
3. Define AIDS and HIV.
4. Explain how the disease is transmitted.
5. Describe and tell how AIDS symptoms differ from regular flu symptoms.
6. [2nd lesson] Explain what the HIV antibody test measures in a person.
7. Explain three ways one can prevent contracting AIDS.

Grades 11 and 12 (16 years and older)

1. Define AIDS and HIV virus.
2. Explain the meaning of the AIDS antibody test.
3. List three kinds of risky behavior for contracting AIDS.

[2nd day]

4. Identify two common myths about the transmission of AIDS.
5. Explain why donating blood is not and has not been a way for HIV to be transmitted in the U.S.
6. Explain how a healthy-looking person can transmit HIV.
7. List three symptoms of the HIV virus.
8. Describe three methods of HIV infection.
9. List two local resources where more information about AIDS can be found.

Although "readiness for sex" is mentioned and students are given a reminder that they can say "no," little is done either to help students identify and anticipate situations where they may experience sexual pressure or to equip them experientially with assertive tools to say "no" effectively. Students are likely to be given a very false sense of security by virtue of the curriculum's consistent and explicit advocacy of condom use "if you decide to become sexually active."

What emerges from the preceding survey of content and strategies currently in place with respect to Sex/AIDS Education is the same ineffective pattern observed on a smaller scale by the staff of the Teen Services Program in Atlanta:

- most programs in place are knowledge-based;
- they employ explicit/implicit adult decision-making strategies;
- they employ strategies inconsistent with the psychological development of adolescents;
- they have failed to address the most important expressed need of adolescents: resisting pressure to engage in sexual activity.

In effect, at the national, state and local levels, educators have consistently adopted the least effective medical and educational strategies to stop the spread of AIDS among adolescents, to reduce the levels of sexual activity, teenage pregnancy and transmission of STD's.

Alternative Sexuality Education Programs

Adolescent Pregnancy Care and Prevention Program
123 N. Avenue N.
Lubbock, TX 79401

Family Life/Human Sexuality Education Curriculum
Family Life Education Department
St. Margaret's Hospital for Women
Boston, MA 02125

Postponing Sexual Involvement
Grady Memorial Hospital
80 Butter Street, S.E.
Atlanta, GA 30335

Rainbow
Providence Health Foundation
4520 12th Street, N.E.
Washington, D.C. 20017

Sex Respect
Respect Incorporated
P.O. Box 5871
Kankakee, IL 60902

Values and Choices
Search Institute
122 W. Franklin St.
Minneapolis, MN 55404

Sexuality, Commitment and Family
Teen-AID, Inc.
W. 22 Mission
Spokane, WA 99201

Notes

1. AIDS Newsletter, Massachusetts Department of Public Health, November 1991.

2. Hein, K., M.D., "Adolescent Acquired Immunodeficiency Syndrome," *American Journal of Diseases of Children,* Vol. 144, January 1990, p. 47.

3. AIDS Newsletter, Massachusetts Department of Public Health, November 1991.

4. AIDS Newsletter, Massachusetts Department of Public Health, February 1991.

5. AIDS Newsletter, Massachusetts Department of Public Health, November 1991.

6. 1990 Statistical Abstract of the United States, p. 12.

7. AIDS Newsletter, Massachusetts Department of Public Health, November 1991.

8. Ibid.

9. Ibid.

10. Hein, K., M.D., "Lessons from New York City on HIV/AIDS in Adolescents," *New York State Journal of Medicine,* March 1990, p. 143.

11. AIDS Newsletter, Massachusetts Department of Public Health, November 1991.

12. Hein, K., M.D., "Lessons from New York City on HIV/AIDS in Adolescents," *New York State Journal of Medicine,* March 1990, p. 143.

13. Zelnick, M., and Kantner, J.F., "Sexual Activity, Contraceptive Use and Pregnancy Among Metropolitan Area Teenagers: 1971-1979," *Family Planning Perspectives,* 1980, 12:230-231, 233-237.

14. Vermund, S.H., et. al., "Acquired Immune Deficiency Among Adolescents: Case Surveillance in New York City and the Rest of the United States," *American Journal of Diseases of Children,* 1989, 143:1220-1225 (as cited in 10).

15. Novello, A., "A Report of the Secretary's Work Group of Pediatric HIV Infection and Disease," Department of Health and Human Services, November 1988, pp. 17-20 (as cited in 10).

16. Hein, K., M.D., "AIDS in Adolescents: A Rationale for Concern," *New York State Journal of Medicine,* 1987, 87:5, p. 295.

17. Hein, K., M.D. "Commentary on Adolescent Acquired Immunodeficiency Syndrome: The Next Wave of the Human Immunodeficiency Virus Epidemic?" *Journal of Pediatrics,* 1989, 114:1, p. 147.

18. *Issues in Brief,* Alan Guttmacher Institute, 1985, Vol. 5, No. 4, pp. 2, 3.

19. "Condoms and Sexually Transmitted Diseases...Especially AIDS," HHS Publication FDA 90-4239, p. 7.

20. Ibid.

21. Interview with Dr. C. Everett Koop, *USA Today,* September 18, 1987.

22. Wellings, K., "AIDS and the Condom," *British Medical Journal,* 1986, Vol. 293, p. 1259.

23. Goerdent, J., M.D., "What Is Safe Sex?" *New England Journal of Medicine,* 197, Vol. 316, No. 21, pp. 1339-1342.

24. Fischl, M., M.D., "Evaluation of Heterosexual Partners, Children and Household Contacts of Adults with AIDS," *Journal of the American Medical Association,* 197, 257:640-644.

25. "Condoms and Sexually Transmitted Diseases...Especially AIDS," HHS Publication FDA 90-4239.

26. Ibid.

27. Harris and Associates Survey "American Teens Speak: Sex, Myths, TV and Birth Control," Conducted for Planned Parenthood, 1986, p. 26.

28. Olsen, J., and Weed, S., "Effects of Family Planning Programs for Teenagers on Adolescent Births and Pregnancy Rates" and "Effect of Family Planning Programs on Teenage Pregnancy – Replication and Extension," *Family Perspective,* 1986, 20:3.

29. Harris and Associates Survey "American Teens Speak: Sex, Myths, TV and Birth Control," Conducted for Planned Parenthood, 1986, pp. 45, 53.

30. Ibid., p. 60.

31. Dawson, D., "The Effect of Sex Education on Adolescent Behavior," *Family Planning Perspectives,* 1986, 18:4, p. 66.

32. Marsiglio, W., and Mott, F., "The Impact of Sex Education on Sexual Activity, Contraceptive Use and Premarital Pregnancy Among American Teenagers," *Family Planning Perspectives,* 1986, 18:4, pp. 158, 159.

33. Garris, L., et. al., "The Relationship Between Oral Contraceptives and Adolescent Sexual Behavior," *The Journal of Sex Research,* 1976, p. 138; Reichelt, P., "Changes in Sexual Behavior Among Unmarried Teenage Women Utilizing Oral Contraception," *Journal of Population,* 1978, p. 61.

34. Ibid., p. 6.

35. Ibid., p. 9.

36. Zabin, L., et. al., "Evaluation of a Pregnancy Prevention Program for Urban Teenagers," *Family Planning Perspectives,* 1986, 18:3, p. 119.

37. Kegeles, S., et. al., "Sexually Active Adolescents and Condoms: Changes in One Year in Knowledge, Attitude and Use," *American Journal of Public Health,* 1988, 78:4, p. 460.

38. Harris and Associates Survey "American Teens Speak: Sex, Myths, TV and Birth Control," Conducted for Planned Parenthood, 1986, p. 28.

39. Ibid.

40. Kirby, D., et. al., "Six School-Based Clinics: Their Reproductive Health Services and Impact on Sexual Behavior," *Family Planning Perspectives,* 1991, 23:1, p. 13.

41. Harris and Associates Survey "American Teens Speak: Sex, Myths, TV

and Birth Control," Conducted for Planned Parenthood, 1986, p. 64.

42. McAnarney, E., and Hendee, W., "Adolescent Pregnancy and Its Consequences," *Journal of the American Medical Association,* 1989, 262:1, p. 74.

43. Ginsberg, H., and Opper, S., *Piaget's Book of Intellectual Development,* New Jersey, Prentice-Hall, 1969; Chapman, R. H., "The Development of Children's Understanding of Proportions," *Child Development,* 1975, 46:141-148.

44. McAnarney, E., and Hendee, W., "Adolescent Pregnancy and Its Consequences," *Journal of the American Medical Association,* 1989, 262:1, p. 74.

45. Howard, M., and McCabe, J., "Helping Teenagers Postpone Sexual Involvement," *Family Planning Perspectives,* 1990, 22:1, p. 21.

46. Stark, E., "Young, Innocent and Pregnant," *Psychology Today,* October 1986, p. 30.

47. Moore and Burt, "Private Crisis, Public Cost, 1982" (as cited by the Task Force on Pregnant and Parenting Teenagers in Massachusetts, 1986, pp. 18-20).

48. Young, M., "The Planned Parenthood Poll: A Secondary Analysis of National Data," paper presented before the American Alliance for Health, Physical Recreation and Dance, April 1988 (as cited in 45).

49. "How Effective Is AIDS Education?" Office of Technology Assessment, Jane E. Sisk, Study Director, June 1988, p. 34.

50. Stark, E., "Young, Innocent and Pregnant," *Psychology Today,* October 1986, p. 30.

51. Ibid.

52. The Report of the Task Force on Pregnant and Parenting Teenagers in Massachusetts, 1986, pp. 18-20.

53. Moore and Burt, "Private Crisis, Public Cost, 1982" (as cited by the Task Force on Pregnant and Parenting Teenagers in Massachusetts, 1986).

54. The Report of the Task Force on Pregnant and Parenting Teenagers in Massachusetts, 1986, pp. 18-20.

55. Assessment of the School-Based Health Clinics, Welfare Research, Inc., May 13, 1987, p. 25.

56. Orr, D., et. al., "Premature Sexual Activity as an Indicator of Psychosocial Risk," *Pediatrics,* 1991, 87:2, p. 144.

57. Stark, E., "Young, Innocent and Pregnant," *Psychology Today,* October 1986, p. 30.

58. The Report of the Task Force on Pregnant and Parenting Teenagers in Massachusetts, 1986, pp. 18-20.

59. Stark, E., "Young, Innocent and Pregnant," *Psychology Today,* October 1986, p. 32.

60. Howard, M., and McCabe, J., "Helping Teenagers Postpone Sexual Involvement," *Family Planning Perspectives,* 1990, 22:1, p. 21.

61. Ibid., pp. 21, 22.

62. Ibid.

63. Ibid.

64. Ibid., p. 26.

65. Ibid., p. 22.

66. Harris and Associates Survey "American Teens Speak: Sex, Myths, TV and Birth Control," Conducted for Planned Parenthood, 1986, p. 24.

67. AIDS Newsletter, Massachusetts Department of Public Health, November 1991.

68. Friemuth, V., et. al., *Science, Technology and Human Values,* December, 1987, as cited by P. Cameron in *Exposing the AIDS Scandal,* Huntington House, Inc., 1988, p. 92.

69. Ibid.

70. "AIDS Education: More to Be Done," *The Bay State Teacher,* Spring 1991, 5:1, p. 13.

71. Anderson, J., et. al., "HIV/AIDS Knowledge and Sexual Behavior Among High School Students," *Family Planning Perspectives,* 1990, 22:6, p. 253.

72. Ibid., p. 254.

73. Ibid., p. 254.

74. Sonenstein, F., et. al., "Sexual Activity, Condom Use and AIDS Awareness Among Adolescent Males," *Family Planning Perspectives,* 1989, 21:4, pp. 152, 154.

75. Ibid., pp. 152, 154.

76. Sonenstein, F., et. al., "Sexual Activity, Condom Use and AIDS Awareness Among Adolescent Males," *Family Planning Perspectives,* 1989, 21:4, p. 157.

77. Ibid.

78. Strunin, L., and Hingson, R., "Acquired Immunodeficiency Syndrome and Adolescents: Knowledge, Beliefs, Attitudes and Behaviors," *Pediatrics,* 79:825, 1987; and, Hingson, R., et. al., "AIDS Transmission: Changes in Knowledge and Behaviors Among Adolescents," 1986-1988, *Pediatrics* (forthcoming) (as cited in 74).

79. Sonenstein, F., et. al., "Sexual Activity, Condom Use and AIDS Awareness Among Adolescent Males," *Family Planning Perspectives,* 1989, 21:4, p. 156.

80. Ibid., p. 157.

81. Ibid., p. 158.

82. Olsen, J., and Weed, S., "Effects of Family Planning Programs for Teenagers on Adolescent Births and Pregnancy Rates" and "Effect of Family Planning Programs on Teenage Pregnancy – Replication and Extension," *Family Perspective,* 1986, 20:3.

83. Howard, M., and McCabe, J., "Helping Teenagers Postpone Sexual Involvement," *Family Planning Perspectives,* 1990, 22:1, p. 24.

84. Ibid., p. 24.

85. Ibid., p. 25.

86. Anderson, J., et. al., "HIV/AIDS Knowledge and Sexual Behavior Among High School Students," *Family Planning Perspectives,* 1990, 22:6, p. 254.

87. Howard, M., and McCabe, J., "Helping Teenagers Postpone Sexual Involvement," *Family Planning Perspectives,* 1990, 22:1, p. 26.

88. Harris and Associates Survey "American Teens Speak: Sex, Myths, TV and Birth Control," Conducted for Planned Parenthood, 1986, p. 24.

89. Freeman, P., "Risky Business," *People,* 1990, 34:18, p. 56.

90. Harris and Associates Survey "American Teens Speak: Sex, Myths, TV and Birth Control," Conducted for Planned Parenthood, 1986, p. 25.

91. Ibid., pp. 25, 26.

92. Howard, M., and McCabe, J., "Helping Teenagers Postpone Sexual Involvement," *Family Planning Perspectives,* 1990, 22:1, p. 23.

93. Ibid.

94. Ibid., pp. 22, 24.

95. Harris and Associates Survey "American Teens Speak: Sex, Myths, TV and Birth Control," Conducted for Planned Parenthood, 1986, p. 71.

96. Ibid., p. 26.

97. Howard, M., and McCabe, J., "Helping Teenagers Postpone Sexual Involvement," *Family Planning Perspectives,* 1990, 22:1, p. 26.

98. Kirby, D., et. al., "Six School-Based Clinics: Their Reproductive Health Services and Impact on Sexual Behavior," *Family Planning Perspectives,* 1991, 23:1, p. 13.

99. Orr, D., et. al., "Premature Sexual Activity as an Indicator of Psychosocial Risk," *Pediatrics,* 1991, 87:2, p. 144.

100. Harris and Associates Survey "American Teens Speak: Sex, Myths, TV and Birth Control," Conducted for Planned Parenthood, 1986, pp. 22, 23.

101. Ibid., p. 68.

102. Ibid., p. 60.

103. Assessment of the School-Based Health Clinics, Welfare Research, Inc., May 13, 1987, p. 25.

104. Hein, K., M.D., "AIDS in Adolescents: A Rationale for Concern," *New York State Journal of Medicine,* 1987, 87:5, p. 29.

105. Orr, D., et. al., "Premature Sexual Activity as an Indicator of Psychosocial Risk," *Pediatrics,* 1991, 87:2, p. 144.

106. Kenney, A., "Teen Pregnancy: An Issue for Schools," *Phi Delta Kappan,* 1987, p. 730.

107. Conont, J., et. al., "How to Talk About Sex," *Newsweek,* February 16, 1987, p. 68.

108. The Report of the Task Force on Pregnant and Parenting Teenagers in Massachusetts, 1986, pp. 18-20.

109. Harris and Associates Survey "American Teens Speak: Sex, Myths, TV and Birth Control," Conducted for Planned Parenthood, 1986, p. 16.

110. Dawson, D., "The Effect of Sex Education on Adolescent Behavior," *Family Planning Perspectives,* 1986, 18:4, p. 166.

111. Harris and Associates Survey "American Teens Speak: Sex, Myths, TV and Birth Control," Conducted for Planned Parenthood, 1986, pp. 41-44.

112. Ibid., p. 60, by calculation.

113. Dawson, D., "The Effect of Sex Education on Adolescent Behavior," *Family Planning Perspectives,* 1986, 18:4, p. 166.

114. Harris and Associates Survey "American Teens Speak: Sex, Myths, TV and Birth Control," Conducted for Planned Parenthood, 1986, p. 16.

115. Marsiglio, W., and Mott, F., "The Impact of Sexual Activity, Contraceptive Use and Premarital Pregnancy Among American Teenagers," *Family Planning Perspectives,* 1986, 18:4, p. 151.

116. Frye, J., "Sex in the Boston Public Schools," *The Student Voice,* December, 1987.

117. Stark, E., "Young, Innocent and Pregnant," *Psychology Today,* October 1986, p. 33.

118. Harris and Associates Survey "American Teens Speak: Sex, Myths, TV and Birth Control," Conducted for Planned Parenthood, 1986, p. 16.

119. Dawson, D., "The Effect of Sex Education on Adolescent Behavior," *Family Planning Perspectives,* 1986, 18:4, p. 166.

120. Harris and Associates Survey "American Teens Speak: Sex, Myths, TV and Birth Control," Conducted for Planned Parenthood, 1986, p. 16.

121. Kenney, A., "Teen Pregnancy: An Issue for Schools," *Phi Delta Kappan,* 1987, p. 730.

122. The Report of the Task Force on Pregnant and Parenting Teenagers in Massachusetts, 1986, pp. 18-20.

123. "Condoms to Curb AIDS Endorsed at House Hearing," *International Medical News,* 1987, 20:8.

124. Hein, K., M.D., "Commentary on Adolescent Acquired Immunodeficiency Syndrome: The Next Wave of the Human Immunodeficiency Virus Epidemic?" *The Journal of Pediatrics,* 1989, 114:1, p. 145.

125. Harris and Associates Survey "American Teens Speak: Sex, Myths, TV and Birth Control," Conducted for Planned Parenthood, 1986, pp. 15, 16.

126. Howard, M., and McCabe, J., "Helping Teenagers Postpone Sexual Involvement," *Family Planning Perspectives,* 1990, 22:1, p. 23.

127. "Teen Pregnancy: What Is Being Done? A State By State Look," Minority Report of Select Committee on Children, Youth and Families, December 1985, Tables 7 and 8.

128. Howard, M., and McCabe, J., "Helping Teenagers Postpone Sexual Involvement," *Family Planning Perspectives,* 1990, 22:1, p. 24.

129. Sonenstein, F., and Pittman, K., "The Availability of Sex Education in Large City School Districts," *Family Planning Perspectives,* 1984, 16:1, p. 19.

130. Harris and Associates Survey "American Teens Speak: Sex, Myths, TV and Birth Control," Conducted for Planned Parenthood, 1986, pp. 47, 52.

131. Forrest, J., and Silverman, J., "What Public School Teachers Teach About Preventing Pregnancy, AIDS and Sexually Transmitted Diseases," *Family Planning Perspectives,* 1989, 21:2, p. 65.

132. Ibid.

133. Ibid., p. 68.

134. Sonenstein, F., and Pittman, K., "The Availability of Sex Education in Large City School Districts," *Family Planning Perspectives,* 1984, 16:1, p. 19.

135. Ibid.

136. Ibid., p. 68.

137. Ibid., p. 69.

138. Ibid., p. 70.

139. Ibid., p. 68.

140. Ibid., p. 68.

141. Ibid., p. 68.

142. Ibid., p. 69.

143. Ibid., p. 67.

144. Ibid., p. 67.

145. Sonenstein, F., and Pittman, K., "The Availability of Sex Education in Large City School Districts," *Family Planning Perspectives,* 1984, 16:1, p. 21.

146. Ibid., p. 69.

147. Kenney, A., et. al., "Sex Education and AIDS Education in the Schools: What States and Large School Districts Are Doing," *Family Planning Perspectives,* 1989, 21:2, p. 63.

148. Forrest, J., and Silverman, J., "What Public School Teachers Teach About Preventing Pregnancy, AIDS and Sexually Transmitted Diseases," *Family Planning Perspectives,* 1989, 21:2, p. 70.

149. Ibid., p. 68.

150. Ibid., p. 70.

151. Kenney, A., et. al., "Sex Education and AIDS Education in the Schools: What States and Large School Districts Are Doing," *Family Planning Perspectives,* 1989, 21:2, p. 63.

152. Forrest, J., and Silverman, J., "What Public School Teachers Teach About Preventing Pregnancy, AIDS and Sexually Transmitted Diseases," *Family Planning Perspectives,* 1989, 21:2, p. 65.

153. Ibid., p. 70.

154. Ibid., p. 67.

155. Ibid., p. 65.

156. Ibid., p. 70.

157. Kirby, D., et. al., "Six School-Based Clinics: Their Reproductive Health Services and Impact on Sexual Behavior," *Family Planning Perspectives,* 1991, 23:1, p. 6.

158. Ibid.

159. "Courage and Condoms," *The Boston Globe,* March 11, 1991.

160. Harris and Associates Survey "American Teens Speak: Sex, Myths,

TV and Birth Control," Conducted for Planned Parenthood, 1986, p. 71.

161. Ibid., p. 71.

162. Ibid., p. 71.

163. Sonenstein, F., and Pittman, K., "The Availability of Sex Education in Large City School Districts," *Family Planning Perspectives,* 1984, 16:1, p. 22.

164. Ibid., p. 23.

165. Ibid., p. 23.

166. Ibid., p. 22.

167. "AIDS Education: More to Be Done," *The Bay State Teacher,* Spring 1991, 5:1, p. 13.

168. Ibid.

169. Ibid.

170. Ibid.

171. Kenney, A., et. al., "Sex Education and AIDS Education in the Schools: What States and Large School Districts Are Doing," *Family Planning Perspectives,* 1989, 21:2, p. 59.

172. *Learn and Live—A Teaching Guide on AIDS Prevention,* Massachusetts Deptartment of Public Health/Education, August 1987.

173. "AIDS Education: More to Be Done," *The Bay State Teacher,* Spring 1991, 5:1, p. 13.

174. Boston Public Schools High School Health Education Objectives, 1985, p. 78.

175. Boston Public Schools Middle School Health Education Objectives, 1985, pp. 71-78.

176. Boston Public Schools High School Health Education Objectives, 1985, pp. 78-90.

177. Clark, K., et. al., *Two Lesson Plans for AIDS Education for 7th and 8th Grades,* 1988; Cohen S., et. al., *Two Lesson Plans for AIDS Education for 9th and 10th Grades,* 1988; Banks, B., et. al., *Two Lesson Plans for AIDS Education for 11th and 12th Grades,* 1988; Boston Public Schools.